"This is a long-awaited book written s̶p̶____ ̶f̶o̶r̶ ̶p̶a̶t̶i̶e̶n̶t̶s̶ ̶s̶a̶i̶l̶i̶n̶g̶ through the cancer journey, and is an invaluable resource for them to empower themselves in their cancer care."

—**Simon S. Lo, MB, ChB, FACR**, professor and vice-chair for strategic planning of radiation oncology at the University of Washington School of Medicine, and internationally renowned expert in stereotactic radiation delivery and neurologic radiation oncology

"David Palma has developed a refreshing resource for patients who must endure the complicated journey that comes with the diagnosis of cancer. He highlights what questions to ask, why certain tests are done, and where to look for potential mistakes that can affect their outcomes."

—**Drew Moghanaki, MD, MPH**, director of clinical radiation oncology research at Hunter Holmes McGuire Veterans Affairs Medical Center

"If you use a guidebook for a journey, you will need *Taking Charge of Cancer* for a cancer journey. Cancer patients are overwhelmed with information related to the diagnosis, and commonly, it is confusing. Palma's 'how to' approach to complex information is surely a brilliant guiding light"

—**Tony Mok, MD**, chair in the department of clinical oncology at the Chinese University of Hong Kong

"David Palma has written a 'how-to' manual that should be considered a must-have book for anyone with cancer. In clear and easily readable prose, Palma helps patients and their family members navigate the unfamiliar territory in which they find themselves after receiving a diagnosis of malignancy. With a combination of illustrative patient stories and well-explained medical evidence, the book provides authoritative guidance in a general sense, and also specific advice on where to find more information on an individual patient's particular situation. I will recommend it to my patients and to my own family and friends diagnosed with cancer. I am sure they will gain comfort and reassurance from Palma's thoughtful insights."

— **Brian D. Kavanagh, MD, MPH, FASTRO**, professor and chair in the department of radiation oncology at the University of Colorado Denver School of Medicine

"Palma has provided important advice that is easy to read and understand. It is an essential read for any patient with cancer who is about to undergo any type of cancer therapy."

— **Robert J. Cerfolio, MD, MBA, FACS, FCCP**, chief of thoracic surgery and director of the Lung Cancer Service Line at NYU Langone Cancer Center

Taking Charge
of Cancer

What You Need to Know to Get the Best Treatment

David Palma, MD, PhD

New Harbinger Publications, Inc.

Note to Readers

All patient stories in this book are true. However, to protect anonymity, identifying details have been changed and some stories have been merged into composite stories.

Disclaimer

This book is intended as an information resource for those wishing to know more about the importance of quality cancer care. It is accurate to the best of the author's knowledge and has been written in good faith. It does not provide specific medical advice of any kind. It should not be relied upon for any specific purpose, and no representation or warranty is given regarding its accuracy or completeness. The material is not intended to be a substitute for the advice provided by your doctor or health care providers. You are advised to discuss all issues with your doctor. The final decisions about your medical care should be made between you and your doctor. The author and publisher disclaim all liability related to the use of this book. All opinions provided in this book are solely those of the author and may not represent the opinions of any of his associated institutions or hospitals.

Distributed in Canada by Raincoast Books

Copyright © 2017 by David Palma
New Harbinger Publications, Inc.
5674 Shattuck Avenue
Oakland, CA 94609
www.newharbinger.com

Cover design by Amy Shoup

Edited by Cindy Nixon

All Rights Reserved

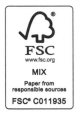

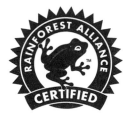

Library of Congress Cataloging-in-Publication Data

19   18   17

10   9   8   7   6   5   4   3   2   1   First Printing

To Cheryl, Kiara, Adam, and William

To Uncle Bob

Contents

Getting World-Class Care

Foreword

If ever there was a time in which a patient's guide to good cancer care was needed, it is now. We are long past the paternalistic age in which cancer patients implicitly trusted their local doctors and did as they were told. That may have been quite sufficient in an era when the treatment options were limited and there was little room for uneven care, but that is not where we are now.

We live in an age of great medical advances, which render a bewildering array of treatment options to patients. We live in an age of hypercommunication, in which information is pouring in from such a variety of sources that it is difficult to curate it, decipher it, and determine what is valuable and what is not. Within this cacophony of information, both doctor and patient can lose control, and the net result has been a very uneven quality of cancer care delivered. The very authoritative Institute of Medicine and a group of very determined researchers at Dartmouth College have documented how patchy the quality of cancer care can be in the United States by geographic region, by hospital, and by physician. Inevitably, this has consequences for patient outcomes and, in particular, the "big two" of survival and quality of life.

I will give you some examples from my own experience as a prostate cancer oncologist. Why is it the case that, in the United States, most men with very mild and early prostate cancers receive aggressive treatment, whereas in the United Kingdom, they are usually observed? Why are these US patients much more likely to undergo surgery in the Pacific Northwest than in New England? Why do reports from very experienced surgeons show low rates of complications, such as urinary incontinence, and yet national studies show rates of the same complications to be very high? The answers, sadly, may lie in dark places. Physicians prefer to do what they do. If a surgeon sees a patient first, then surgery may be the only treatment offered. Surgeons who perform an operation infrequently will not do it as well as those who work in "high-volume" centers. The payment structure in some health care systems may incentivize physicians to use one treatment over another, perfectly good, alternative treatment.

These are problems on the physician side, but what influences good care on the patient side? Firstly, patients may simply ask no questions and seek no confirmation of the initial recommendation. Or perhaps they seek therapies promoted in the media, not realizing that the evidence supporting their use may be very thin. The media always needs good health news stories in its dual role as informer and entertainer, frequently presenting premature data with hyperbolic claims of "miracle cures." Alternative therapies abound in prostate cancer, and although few have strong evidence to support them, there is everything out there from a gigantic, unregulated nutritional supplement industry to a deafening Internet buzz promoting these therapies. More than 50 percent of prostate cancer patients are taking a supplement or altering their diet in response to this.

A few years ago, I had a patient with a tiny prostate cancer that did not threaten him at all and really should have been left alone. He understood this and planned to simply be observed, but he couldn't resist the siren call of Chinese herbs. Well, what's the harm? These he brewed and drank in enormous quantity and concentration with the result that his liver stopped working and he needed a liver transplant. What was worse, in order to be on a waiting list for a precious donor liver, he had to have no other major illnesses and, specifically, he had to be free of any cancer. Thus, I needed to treat his prostate cancer in order to allow him to receive his transplant, which he wouldn't have needed if he hadn't taken the Chinese herbs that he never needed in the first place!

This is a dramatic example, but it does show how difficult it can be for patients to sort the wheat from the chaff, especially if they try to do it alone. I may think of myself as an educated individual, but if I had a legal problem or a plumbing problem, I would be at the mercy of others. Patients diagnosed with cancer are no different and in some ways even more challenged because the consequences can be so serious.

The best defense for someone newly diagnosed with cancer is to take a deep breath and call a time-out. Ask questions, get different opinions, read wisely, and then, after discussion with family and friends, make thoughtful, informed decisions. This, alas, is easier said than done. What questions should you ask? Where can you find reliable information? How do you distinguish fact from fiction? How do you tell a competent physician from a self-promoter? Most doctors practice in good faith, but they often don't know what they don't know and have biases bred from the quirks of their training and experience. A solo practitioner may be good but has less oversight than someone who works in teams. A young physician may lack experience, but an older one may not have kept up.

The rise of the multidisciplinary cancer clinic is one of the great quality advances in modern cancer care. Having physicians from different specialties in the same room, together with the patient, allows for coordination of complex care while at the same time keeping everyone honest. It is difficult for a physician to understate the side effects of his or her treatment when colleagues are present.

When you go to a new city in a different land where you don't speak the language, you need a guidebook, a translator, and a map. David Palma's book is all three. It leads the patient by the hand through this complicated process, stopping to explain and point out the scenery and the traps on the way. This is a land where getting lost and making bad decisions can have consequences either for the rest of your life or, simply, for your life. There is no room for error. In clear language and with examples from his own practice, Dr. Palma does what all physicians, in an ideal world, would like to do. If you have recently been diagnosed with cancer, take time with this book and take time with your decisions. There is no better advice that I can give you.

—Anthony Zietman, MD
October 2016

Introduction

CHAPTER 1

Taking Charge Can Improve Your Chances

Today's cancer patients are better informed than ever before. Many patients come to their doctor equipped with a stack of literature and a good understanding of their diagnosis and treatment. But a crucial component is missing.

Most patients have no idea that the quality of their treatment is a key factor that can influence their survival. Making matters worse is the fact that even if patients were aware of this issue, they don't have the tools to evaluate whether their team is providing top-notch care. When a patient receives recommendations from her doctor, it is very difficult to know if those recommendations are good ones. In many instances, she may never know if her doctor has made a critical mistake.

Delivering cancer treatment to patients is very complex. Treating cancer is not like following a simple recipe, where mixing the same ingredients in any kitchen gives the same results. Cancer care for a single patient requires decisions from numerous professionals to dispense treatments that are potentially life-saving, but also potentially dangerous and life-threatening. The chances of cure and survival for any given patient depend on the expertise of the cancer team and whether procedures are in place to ensure that cancer care is delivered properly.

How important is the quality of cancer treatment? The numbers are dramatic. For a patient undergoing cancer surgery, the risk of dying from surgery can be reduced substantially—in some cases, reduced by more than half—depending on the choice of surgeon and hospital.[1] For a patient undergoing radiation, the risk of dying from cancer or treatment can be nearly cut in half with similar choices.[2] These differences are well studied and known to doctors and researchers, but this information has not reached the public.

Big medical mistakes sometimes make headlines. In 2015, a doctor in Michigan was stripped of his license and sentenced to decades in jail for giving chemotherapy to patients who didn't even have cancer and for giving patients with cancer the wrong chemotherapy. Several North American radiation centers gave the wrong doses of radiation. These big mistakes—gross negligence in some cases—can result in serious harm.* But smaller errors, those that more easily fly under the radar and might not make headlines, can also have a major impact on individual patients. A forgotten test result, an incorrect dose of a drug, a treatment recommendation that goes against currently accepted guidelines—any of these can have serious consequences.

Richard Meyer was almost one of those patients. When I met him, he was a healthy single guy in his forties who had just been diagnosed with cancer. Richard had developed painless lumps in his neck a few months prior, and the largest was the size of a golf ball. A doctor had put a needle into a lump to take a *biopsy* (a sample of tissue), and the specimen showed cancer. The lumps were actually enlarged lymph nodes that had filled with cancer.** The cancer had

---

* To read more about the doctor in Michigan and the radiation errors, go to http://www.qualitycancertreatment.com/a01.

** *Lymph nodes* are small glands in the body that usually fight infection, but many cancers use them as a route of spread.

traveled to those lymph nodes from somewhere else, but doctors weren't sure exactly where.

In a situation like this, doctors go looking to find out where the cancer has come from. Sometimes we find the location, and sometimes we don't. Either way, knowing where the cancer came from—or ruling out possible sources—has an enormous impact on the treatment. If we find where the tumor is from, then the treatment is quite different than if the original source remains undiscovered.

Richard's doctors checked his chest and looked in his nose, mouth, and throat, but they couldn't find the original source of cancer. They even took biopsies from a few locations where the tumor could have come from, but those biopsy samples didn't show any cancer. So they chalked it up to a situation in which the original tumor can't be found. Richard's recommended treatment—radiation with chemotherapy—was all set to start.

But unbeknownst to Richard, he was being treated at a hospital that did not specialize in treating his type of cancer. Just before he started that treatment, one of his doctors had a realization: Richard's case was missing something important. For all major types of cancer, there are widely available guidelines that are designed to help make sure that physicians are taking the correct approaches to diagnosis and treatment. These guidelines are written by panels of experts and updated frequently, and they represent the best recommendations for cancer treatment. Treatment guidelines recommend that all patients with head and neck cancers like Richard's be seen by a surgeon specializing in treating such cancers.* But Richard hadn't seen such a surgeon.

Treatment was put on hold. He was sent to a surgeon at the hospital where I work. The surgeon did a standard assessment. He talked to Richard to hear his story, reviewed the scans, felt Richard's neck

---

* You will learn to access guidelines later in this book.

for lumps, and looked in his mouth. Then he passed a small tube with a camera up his nose to look inside, repeating a procedure that had already been done by the other doctors.

And he found it. The cancer was subtle but unmistakable, tucked away in the area behind the nasal passages. The surgeon found it because he had an experienced eye and could see a subtle abnormality, having examined and treated thousands of patients with head and neck cancers in his career. A biopsy was taken in the office, and the site of cancer was confirmed.

I met Richard the next day. We designed a new radiation treatment plan for him, including a high dose of radiation targeted to that area where the cancer was now discovered and to the lumps in his neck, and we gave him chemotherapy. The cancer melted away completely.

To this day, more than four years later, Richard's cancer has not returned. But if the original site had not been found, the situation could have been very different. Without knowing where the cancer was, the original doctors may not have delivered enough radiation to get rid of it.

Richard's story teaches us that the quality of cancer treatment varies at different centers and that differences in quality can have a major impact on the chances of cure. Richard's original team did not have the depth of experience that would have made it easier for them to detect the cancer at the back of his nasal passages. They also weren't following established guidelines for assessing a patient before coming up with a treatment plan. One of the doctors caught the error at the last minute, but if Richard had known where to look (as you will learn later in this book), he would have been able to check the guidelines and catch the error himself.

Sometimes errors can be big, but even the small stuff—like ordering the correct tests before treatment—can be important. Studies show that many patients with lung cancer, for example, do not receive the recommended tests to determine the extent of cancer prior to starting treatment. Underscanning patients gives us an incomplete picture of where the cancer could be. Conversely, for women with early breast cancer and men with low-risk prostate cancer, the opposite is happening: patients are being overscanned before treatment.[3] Despite guidelines saying that scans are not needed and studies showing that they will not be helpful, some doctors are ordering them anyway, looking for cancer in places where they are very unlikely to find anything. The problem with this over-scanning is that it wastes time and money, it delays treatment, and these scans can have false positives: red herrings that require even more tests to prove that there is no spread of cancer. If patients had access to treatment guidelines, they could make sure that the correct tests—and only the correct tests—are being done.

Getting quality care is not just about preventing medical errors. We know that other factors besides errors can impact patient outcomes. Quality care includes several things:

- Undergoing the correct tests prior to the start of treatment

- Getting up-to-date recommendations from your doctors that reflect the latest science

- Full disclosure of all the potential benefits and risks of treatment before making a decision, including answering all your questions

- Getting state-of-the-art treatment with appropriate safety mechanisms in place

- Accessing supportive care as needed, including addressing symptoms, side effects, and emotions

- Getting appropriate monitoring after treatment

This book is meant to help you obtain all of these things.

How This Book Works

This book is written as a how-to manual. It is broken into sections and is structured in a way that follows the cancer journey for most patients.

We start with reviewing the basics in the next chapter—the things you need to know to understand cancer, how it can spread, and how it is treated.

We then move on to the part titled Understanding Your Situation, wherein chapters 3 and 4 discuss how to make the most of your first consultation with your cancer doctors and how to obtain and decipher your medical records. These steps are critical to your care, because only when you are fully informed about your situation can you make sure you are getting the best treatment.

In the next section, Evaluating Your Doctor's Recommendations (chapters 5–8), you will learn how doctors use evidence to decide which treatments are best, how controversies can erupt when the data is not clear, and how doctors can become biased in their recommendations. You will learn how to get second opinions, how to double-check if the recommendations made by your doctors are in keeping with accepted treatment guidelines, and if there are other treatment options you should be considering.

The second half of the book is dedicated to ensuring you receive world-class treatment. It will help you to evaluate whether the surgery, radiation, and/or chemotherapy that are offered to you will be provided in the highest-caliber manner. We will discuss the option of joining a clinical trial and why trials can be a good idea in many cases. We will then move on to two other situations: what to do once treatment is done and things to consider when there is no cure. After these discussions, I review many of the myths and truths about cancer. Many patients feel overwhelmed by the amount of advice they get—sometimes unsolicited—about possible treatments for their cancer, and this chapter can help. Chapter 15 contains the *Taking Charge of Cancer* Patient Checklist, which allows you to easily review the main items in this book.

This book also provides you with an online Patient Toolkit, which you can access at http://www.qualitycancertreatment.com/ toolkit. The toolkit contains helpful resources, such as a spreadsheet to keep track of your medical records (with a video explaining how to use it), along with several other important how-to videos.

As we go through the book, I'll also provide you with useful links, either as footnotes at the bottom of the page or in the resources section at the end of select chapters. Because some of the links are long strings of text, in some cases, I've given you a short link through the Quality Cancer Treatment website (http://www.qualitycancer treatment.com) instead. If there is a printed link in this book to an external site that is no longer working by the time you read this, you can check the website for a new link for that resource (at http://www. qualitycancertreatment.com/links).

For most people, reading the chapters in order makes the most sense, because the book's progression parallels the time-course of their diagnosis and treatment. But if you are at a specific phase in your treatment—for example, about to have surgery—you will find it useful to start with the chapters that are most pertinent to you and read the rest later.

Why I Wrote This Book

The current approach for most patients with cancer is to just learn generic information about their type of cancer and its treatment options. For a woman with breast cancer, for instance, she will learn what breast cancer is, how it's diagnosed, and how it's treated— usually with surgery and maybe some radiation, chemotherapy, or other drugs. This approach is not enough.

This book is meant to help you take the next step, learning about what constitutes good treatment and what does not. By becoming aware of what constitutes top-notch treatment, you and other patients can then choose to go to the hospitals that provide it or you can ask your doctors to take the steps necessary to provide good care. If enough patients demand the very best care, more doctors will provide it, and the system will be improved for everyone.

In our information-overloaded world, it's important to start with a healthy skepticism of anything you read. Cancer information is everywhere—on the Internet, in bookstores, and sometimes in your e-mail inbox. Some of the information you'll find elsewhere is well written and extremely valuable (I will point you to some of these good sources), but some of the advice is bogus. It can be hard to know what to believe. When reading anything medical-related, ask yourself: *Who wrote this, what is their background, what might their motives be, and why should I believe them?* We will talk about how to distinguish cancer truths from myths later on in chapter 15. But before reading beyond this chapter, you need to ask yourself: *Why should I trust the information written in this book?*

There are several very good reasons. First, my biography (at the end of this book) shows that I have the right background and training and that I'm an expert in this field. I have advanced degrees and awards from some excellent universities. I'm a *radiation oncologist*—a doctor who treats cancer with radiation—and I am a cancer researcher. I have written or cowritten more than 100 research papers, and I lead several important clinical trials. I'm an invited lecturer or teacher at mainstream cancer conferences around the world. So the background fits.

Second, the information presented in this book is based on scientific studies. At the end of the book, I provide references (corresponding to the superscript note numbers throughout the book) that anyone can double-check for accuracy. This is your assurance that my arguments are based on facts. You can go back to the original studies and read them.

Third, you should know that I'm not an "antiestablishment" activist. I'm not going to suggest anything that goes against science. Do not abandon mainstream medicine and choose vitamin C as the treatment for your cancer. A decision like that could be suicidal (we'll discuss this later in the book). Rather, I am a staunch supporter of our best establishments: the cancer centers that deliver world-class care, the organizations that support cancer research, those that write treatment guidelines, and the websites and books that provide accurate patient information. My goal is that *every* patient receives the world-class care that these very best centers and doctors already provide.

I'm not a lone wolf in my belief that many patients aren't getting the highest-quality care. In 1999, the Institute of Medicine (recently renamed the National Academy of Medicine) produced a comprehensive report called *Ensuring Quality Cancer Care*. The report concluded that "for many Americans with cancer, there is a wide gulf between what could be construed as the ideal and the reality of their experience with cancer care." It goes on to state that "some individuals with cancer do not receive care known to be effective for their condition. The magnitude of the problem is not known, but the National Cancer Policy Board believes it is substantial."[4] The report made several recommendations on how cancer care could be improved, some of which are reflected in this book. A follow-up report published in 2012 concluded that while the 1999 report has led to improvements, "it is clear that some cancer patients are not receiving ideal care despite these efforts."[5]

This is a view shared by Dr. Vincent DeVita Jr., probably the most esteemed medical oncologist in the United States (*medical oncologists* are doctors who deliver chemotherapy). He pioneered the use of chemotherapy for the treatment of Hodgkin's lymphoma, one of the first cancers to be cured with chemotherapy. He's been the director of the National Cancer Institute and chief physician at Memorial Sloan Kettering Cancer Center. He wrote the textbook that has been used for decades as the premier source of information for oncologists around the world. His recent book, *The Death of Cancer*, describes the successes in cancer research over the past 40 years, but it also lays bare some unflattering problems, including physician biases, infighting, and difficulty ensuring that patients get good-quality care. DeVita writes: "Most people think that cancer centers are comprehensive, one-stop-shopping cancer facilities. Whatever type of cancer you have, they can handle every aspect of it. But the truth is, they can't." He goes on to say: "Cancer centers don't especially want patients to know about their deficiencies" and "If you are diagnosed with a cancer that might be fatal, you cannot assume that the nearest cancer center has the necessary expertise for your particular cancer."[6]

I wrote this book because I realized that something was fundamentally unfair. As an oncologist, I'm often asked for advice on behalf of family or friends who have been recently diagnosed with cancer. What do I tell them? I advise them to obtain their medical records, I help to decipher them, I double-check that the recommendations and treatments are correct, and I make sure the treatment is given at a top-notch center. But this is unfair because not everyone has an extra oncologist to double-check their treatment. Patients need the tools to do this themselves, and this book provides these tools.

It might seem daunting to venture into the unknown world of cancer treatment, but the process is relatively straightforward. By delving into the unknown, you can have a positive impact, improving your odds of beating cancer. You might find out that your doctors are doing everything correctly and your treatment is being delivered properly. This will boost your confidence in your team. But you might discover something that leads to a change in your treatment. The time to discover these problems is as early as possible, when issues can still be corrected. The approach taken in this book will put you in the driver's seat of your own cancer treatment.

CHAPTER 2

The Basics

Before we discuss how to take control of your cancer treatment, we need to review some of the basics: what cancer is, how it causes problems, and how we treat it. You'll also learn, in easy-to-understand terms, the meaning of a lot of the basic terms your doctors will use. This material will prepare you to understand everything that follows in the upcoming chapters.

Visiting a doctor can be like going to a foreign country where you don't speak the language. We doctors use technical terms to communicate with one another about medical issues, just as pilots and mechanics each have their own languages. I'm often confused when my mechanic is explaining what needs to be repaired on my car, so it's natural for you to get confused by the terms that doctors use.

Part of taking control of your cancer treatment involves learning the language that oncologists use. You'll need it to understand your own medical records. I'll walk you through much of the lingo as we go through this book, but if you come across a word you don't understand—either here, in your medical records, or elsewhere—there are links to online medical dictionaries at the end of this chapter. They should be sufficient to provide the definition to almost any word you come across.

What Is Cancer?

The human body is made of cells, trillions of them. Each cell is so small that it can be seen only with a microscope. Cells are tiny living balls, all stuck together, and together, they make up our organs and do all of the little jobs that keep our bodies working. Not all are round, though. Some cells are flat, and others look like little cubes. The strangest-shaped cells are our nerve cells, each one looking like a little octopus, with tentacles that reach out to touch other cells and send messages.

Cells have very important functions within the body, and different cells have different jobs. The job of a heart muscle cell is to use energy to contract. Together, millions of these tiny heart muscle cells squeezing and relaxing in unison cause our hearts to beat, pumping blood throughout the body. Meanwhile, nerve cells have a different job. They transmit messages around the body. As you read this, nerve cells at the back of your eyes are sending messages to your brain, providing information about what you see. If you have eaten recently, the cells of your digestive tract are absorbing nutrients into your bloodstream. And during this time, the cells of your immune system are patrolling your body, seeking out and destroying any invaders, such as viruses or bacteria.

Our cells are very carefully programmed, much like a computer would be. Computer programs and cells both do their jobs by following written instructions. A computer program is written by typing out hundreds or thousands of lines of instructions. For a cell, those written instructions are contained in the cell's *deoxyribonucleic acid,* a chemical commonly referred to by its shortened form "DNA."

DNA is an enormous list of instructions. To do their jobs, cells read the parts of the DNA that are meant for them. The muscle cells read the parts of the DNA that are needed for muscle cells to do their job, while the nerve cells read the parts of the DNA that are needed for nerve cells.

How exactly does this work? In basic terms, within the entire set of DNA, there are thousands of little instructions called "genes." Many of the genes are blueprints for making a protein that can do whatever job the cell needs to get done. Let's say, for example, that you've been going to the gym and working out. Afterward, your muscle cells will try to develop more squeezing power, to make you stronger for next time. A muscle cell will read the genes that tell it how to make more of the proteins that are used to squeeze.* The next time you go to the gym, your muscles will be able to contract a little bit harder because they have more of those proteins.

The lives of our normal cells are very tightly controlled. Most cells spend all their time in one location, just doing their normal job. Those muscle cells in your heart are contracting and relaxing as you read this. As long as they are healthy, those cells will always be well-behaved muscle cells. They are not going to take off and travel somewhere else in your body to do something different. They are also not going to start growing uncontrollably, because their reproduction is also tightly controlled.

When more cells are needed, many cells can divide: one cell becomes two, those two divide again to become four, then eight, sixteen, thirty-two, and so on. But adult cells cannot divide forever, so after a certain number of divisions, they stop. In adults, some cells never divide under normal conditions (like some nerve cells), but many still do. We constantly replace the cells of our skin, digestive tract, and bloodstream. This creation of more cells is carefully

---

* Although it's not too important for the purposes of this book, a more complete picture goes like this: each gene is a blueprint to make *ribonucleic acid,* or "RNA." When a cell wants to read a gene, it copies the message into RNA, and the RNA is a code for how to build whichever proteins the cell needs. DNA also contains other types of instructions, but they are not important for our discussion here.

regulated—once there are enough cells to do the job, cell division stops or slows down.

Even the death of our cells is carefully controlled. Cells can self-destruct—they can end their own lives—when they are damaged or no longer needed. There are instructions in their DNA that tell them how to monitor themselves and how to self-destruct if something is amiss. As an extra safety measure, the "cell police," or *immune system,* is constantly on patrol for renegade cells. The cells of the immune system float around the body looking for misbehaving cells and can kill on sight. This whole process, creating new cells when required and getting rid of damaged or unneeded ones, is crucial to our survival. Cancer arises when this process goes wrong. Cancer is cell growth gone wild.

A normal cell becomes a cancer cell when it doesn't stop dividing and begins to cause problems. In a cancer cell, the DNA has changed—we use the word "mutated"—in a way that gives the cells the wrong instructions. Just like changing a line of code in a computer program can cause the program to do different things, a change in the DNA code can do the same thing for a cell. Mutations can be caused by many things: some occur naturally as we age, but other causes include cigarette smoke, ultraviolet light and other types of radiation, some viruses, and some chemicals. In a cancer cell, the mutations tell the cell to start dividing and not to stop. Instead of staying in the location where it's supposed to be, the cancer cell learns to move, invading other tissues, traveling to lymph nodes, or circulating through the bloodstream to land in other parts of the body to start growing there.

The Hallmarks of Cancer

The development of cancer is more complex than just rogue cells gaining the ability to divide without stopping and travel to other parts of the body. Cancer cells can be different from normal cells in several ways, and these differences are called the "Hallmarks of Cancer."[7] The Hallmarks of Cancer were described by two leaders in cancer biology, Douglas Hanahan, PhD, and Robert Weinberg, PhD. The list of hallmarks is easy to understand, even if you have no scientific background, and can help you grasp exactly what a cancer cell does and why doctors design some treatments the way they do.

The Hallmarks of Cancer tell us that cancer cells are programmed to divide. Our normal cells can divide only a limited number of times, but cancer cells can keep dividing forever. Cancer cells are considered immortal unless treated. Cancer cells avoid or ignore signals that tell them to stop dividing, and they also ignore signals to self-destruct. They find ways to hide from the immune system. Since cancer cells need nutrients just like any other cells, they can send out signals that recruit blood vessels to bring those nutrients. They also find new ways of using energy to grow.

Most concerning of all, as mentioned earlier, cancer cells learn to invade normal tissues and can learn to travel to other parts of the body and cause trouble there. Cancer cells also have tricks that can make them increasingly more aggressive and resistant to treatment over time. First, even though cancer cells already have mutations in their DNA, their DNA can be unstable, meaning that more mutations can occur quickly. For example, a cancer cell might quickly develop a mutation that allows it to pump chemotherapy out of the cell, where it can't kill the cancer. Second, cancer cells can cause inflammation—just like a constant irritation—and this inflammation can enable a cancer to become more aggressive.

So, to summarize, the Hallmarks of Cancer include these features:

- Cancer cells can keep dividing forever and are immortal unless treated.

- They avoid or ignore signals to stop dividing or to self-destruct.

- They can recruit blood vessels and use energy in new ways in order to grow.

- They can hide from the immune system.

- They can invade normal tissues and travel to other parts of the body.

- Because of their unstable DNA and the inflammation they cause, they can become more aggressive over time.

Cancer Is Not a Single Disease

We talk of "cancer" as being a single disease, but it is not. Cancer is actually hundreds of different diseases under one label. There are many, many types of cancers, including lung, breast, prostate, colon, skin, stomach, brain, and bone cancers. A cancer can arise from almost any cell in the body. Some cancers are common— such as lung, prostate, breast, and colon—and some are rare, like cancers of the muscles or nerves. All of these different types of cancers behave differently, and they respond differently to treatment. A breast cancer has a different set of genetic instructions than a lung cancer or a colon cancer, so it has different patterns of behavior and spread. Even cancers from the same location in the body will often behave differently in different patients, because the exact mutations can be different.

Even more striking, cancer cells *within the same patient* can be different from one another. If a surgeon removes a lung cancer and we decode the DNA in the cells within, we would see that the individual cancer cells can have different mutations and might respond differently to treatment.[8]

18

How Cancer Causes Problems

We've learned that cancer is cell growth gone awry and that cancer cells behave differently from normal cells. Now it becomes easy to understand how cancer can cause problems and how, in some cases, cancer can become life-threatening.

There are three major ways that cancer causes problems. The most obvious way is by growing larger and causing problems in the organ where it arose. Left untreated, a cancer in the colon can grow large enough to block the intestines, a lung cancer can block the airways, and a prostate cancer can make it impossible to pass urine. Even benign tumors can cause some of these problems; although they don't spread to other areas of the body, they can push on important organs.

The second—and more common—way that a cancer causes problems is by traveling through the bloodstream to another organ in the body. The cancer then grows in the new location and can disrupt the function of that organ. For example, a lung cancer can travel to the liver and grow there until the liver no longer works properly. In this situation, even though the cancer is no longer in the lung, it is still a lung cancer, because the lung is where it came from originally. This process of traveling to another part of the body is called "metastasis." A cancer that has spread in this way is called a "metastatic cancer." Cancers can travel to the brain, bone, lung, liver, skin, and other locations in the body.

A third way that a cancer can cause problems is by releasing chemicals, or hormones, into the bloodstream that can have unwanted effects. These substances can cause fatigue, decreased appetite and weight loss, or imbalances in our hormonal systems that can be serious. For example, hormones released by some cancer cells lead to very high levels of calcium or very low levels of sodium in the blood.

These complications might sound scary, but fortunately for many patients, these events never happen.

Why is it important to know about these things? These possible problems explain why doctors usually want to treat a cancer as early as possible, since that can prevent irreversible complications. They also explain why we sometimes recommend cancer treatments that can be hard on the body. We don't like to make our patients unwell, but if we give a gentler but less effective treatment, the cancer can come back and cause some of these problems or even be fatal.

How Doctors Know You Have Cancer

Most of the time, to make a diagnosis of cancer, doctors need a sample of the tumor that they can look at under the microscope—from a biopsy. Depending on where the cancer is located, your doctor will choose an appropriate approach to get a sample. For a skin cancer, a biopsy is usually very easy because the cancer is visible. The doctor can cut off a little piece, or the whole thing, using some special instruments. Other times, a needle is used to get a biopsy. For prostate cancer, needles are placed into the prostate (usually through the rectum) to get a sample. For lung cancer, a sample can sometimes be obtained by putting a device with a camera down the windpipe into the lungs, and once the tumor is seen, the doctor can grab a piece. For a colon cancer, the camera goes up into the colon to find the tumor and take a sample.

Regardless of the approach, once a sample is obtained, a *pathologist*—a specific kind of doctor who specializes in looking at tissue samples—will look at it under a microscope and describe what is seen. Sometimes special chemicals or stains are used to better visualize the tumor. The pathologist types up the findings into a written *pathology report*. Since cancer treatment depends on the type of cancer, the pathology report is one of the most important documents in your medical file. It sets the stage for all the treatment recommendations (as you will see in chapter 4), so an error involving a pathology report can lead to major problems.

A few types of cancer can be diagnosed without a biopsy. For some of the cancers of the blood (*leukemias*), just drawing some blood serves as the biopsy because that blood is examined under the microscope. A small number of other cancers can be diagnosed definitively on a blood test, including one type of liver cancer and some cancers of the reproductive organs. But most of the time, a biopsy is needed.

Can doctors diagnose cancers based on imaging tests, such as a *computed tomography* (CT) or *magnetic resonance imaging* (MRI) scan? In some cases, an abnormality seen on a scan is *almost* certainly cancer—the chances that it is cancer may be 95 percent or even higher. But 100 percent certainty usually requires a biopsy. Other things can look like a cancer on a scan, including some kinds of infections. This uncertainty is reflected in the reports we receive from the *radiologist* (the doctor who reviews the scans and issues a report). The radiologist rarely says, "This is a cancer" unless there has already been a biopsy to confirm it. Even in the most suspicious cases, the wording is more nuanced, as in, "This is highly suspicious for cancer" or "Cancer is the most likely diagnosis." Even a scan that is almost 100 percent definitive for cancer won't provide all the information that would result from a biopsy, including the specific type of cancer and sometimes additional information that allows doctors to tailor treatment.

If you have not had a biopsy to confirm that you have cancer, you should ask your doctors: "How are you sure that this is cancer?" If you have had a biopsy, you can get a copy of the pathology report and read it for yourself (we'll discuss this further in chapter 4).

Words to Describe Cancer

When your doctor is discussing your test results, you might hear some new words. Your doctor might describe a "shadow," a "lump," a "spot," or a "tumor." The doctor might use the word "benign" or "malignant." We need to clear up some of the mystery around this lingo.

When a patient undergoes a scan, such as a CT scan or an MRI scan, there might be an abnormality found, something that shouldn't be there. This abnormality could be an area of infection, scarring, an area of cancer, abnormal blood vessels, or several other things. The technical term for an abnormality is a "lesion," but when speaking to patients, we often use less technical terms, calling it a "spot" or a "shadow." If it's big, it might be called a "mass." These terms mean that something is abnormal, but they don't say for sure that it's cancer. If there's a lesion in the liver, it could be one of several things, but not necessarily cancer.

The word "tumor" is used when the abnormality—the lesion—is a collection of growing cells. If it's a tumor, it's not a scar or an infection, and it means that cells are growing. Tumors can be *benign* or *malignant*. Doctors can tell the difference by taking a biopsy.

If the tumor is cancer, then we use the word "malignant." The words "cancer" and "malignant" are interchangeable. If you are told that a biopsy shows malignant cells, it's cancer. Something that is "benign" is not cancer (and therefore also not malignant). Benign tumors cannot spread to other parts of the body like cancers do, and benign tumors usually don't cause serious problems, unless they are pushing on an organ that is critical. So if you have cancer, it's not benign.

Cancer Comes in Stages

The recommended treatment for a patient with cancer is almost always based on two major things: (1) the type of cancer and (2) the *stage*, or the extent of spread.

The type of cancer is determined by looking at the biopsy under the microscope; this can tell us that it's a lung cancer or a breast cancer or some other type of cancer. Lung cancer is treated differently than breast cancer and any other cancer. Even if it is a lung cancer that has spread to the liver, it is still treated like a lung cancer. There can be different types of cancer that arise within each organ, depending on which type of cell the cancer arose from. For example, the vast majority of lung cancers are usually *adenocarcinoma, squamous cell carcinoma,* or *small cell carcinoma.* These are just names for different types of cancers, based on how the cells look under the microscope.

The "stage" of cancer tells doctors whether the cancer has spread anywhere. Most cancers are staged on a scale ranging from I to IV (using Roman numerals). On that scale, stage I usually refers to a small tumor that hasn't invaded very far, grown too big, or traveled anywhere else. Stage IV usually refers to a cancer that has spread through the bloodstream to other parts of the body, and stage II and III are in between, where the tumor is larger than in stage I or has spread to some lymph nodes but not to other organs in the body. The staging system varies for each type of cancer.

The stage conveys very important information to doctors and makes communication easier. For example, if I'm asked to see a patient with stage I lung cancer, I know immediately, even before seeing the patient, which treatment options might be appropriate and which are wrong or harmful. Those options would be completely different for a patient with a different stage of lung cancer.

The stage is critical for determining the treatment path, but most patients don't realize this. Some patients do indeed ask me for their stage, but it's usually one of a list of questions from a handbook, and they just move on to the next question without realizing the importance of the answer I just gave. A better approach would be to ask for the stage, ask why that stage has been assigned, and ask what that stage means in terms of treatment options and outlook. Later on, you will learn how to double-check that you have been assigned the correct stage and then how to check which treatment options are recommended for that stage of cancer.

Fast- and Slow-Growing Cancers

The speed of growth of a cancer can be determined only by looking at two scans over a period of time. Doctors can measure the difference in size between the two scans to get an idea of the speed of growth.

Under the microscope, we can also get an idea of how quickly a cancer is growing and its *grade*, which means how aggressive the cancer appears to be. Faster-growing cancers are high-grade, slower-growing cancers are low-grade, and cancers in between are intermediate-grade. Often the grades have corresponding numbers from 1 to 3 (low to high), and in some cancers, there is a grade 4, which is also considered high-grade.

For some types of cancer, such as breast cancer and prostate cancer, the grade is very important and figures prominently in the treatment decisions. For other types of cancer, such as lung cancer, the grade does not often influence the treatment options.

How Cancer Is Treated

Doctors have three main weapons against cancer. The first is *surgery,* which involves cutting out the tumor, sometimes along with nearby lymph nodes that might contain cancer. The second is *radiation,* an invisible beam that is aimed at the cancer cells. Radiation damages the cells, including the DNA, with the goal of killing them. The immune system then cleans up the dead cells. Surgery and radiation therapy are called "local therapies," because they work only in one location. Surgery is effective only in the area where the surgeon is operating, and radiation treatment works only in the area where the radiation beams hit the cancer cells.*

The third weapon we have is *medications.* These are usually given *intravenously* (into a vein), but they are sometimes taken as pills by mouth. Medications are different than local therapies because they travel through the bloodstream and circulate throughout the body. Because they travel throughout the whole system, they are called *systemic therapy.* Systemic therapy includes drugs known as *chemotherapy,* which tend to also affect normal cells, and newer, more specific tailored drugs that include *targeted agents* (named such because they're designed to better home in on the cancer) and *immunotherapy* (designed to induce the immune system to attack the cancer).

In most cases, systemic therapies by themselves cannot cure a cancer. There are a few exceptions to this rule, like cancers of the immune system (lymphomas and leukemias) and some other types of

---

* Less commonly, other local treatments are available that try to kill the tumor using microwaves, cold, ultrasound, or other approaches. Although radiation is considered a local treatment, in rare cases, the *abscopal effect* can result, which is when radiation to a tumor can alert the immune system that the cancer is there, and the immune system can then attack other locations. The word "abscopal" just means "away from the target." Scientists are working to understand this phenomenon so we can try to use the immune system as our ally.

cancers that are very sensitive to drugs. For the most part, though, some type of local treatment (surgery or radiation) is necessary for a chance at cure.

Measuring the Success of Treatment

"Doc, how will you know if I'm cured after treatment?"

This is probably the most common question I get from patients. As the end of treatment approaches, it's the most natural question. Unfortunately, the answer is not very satisfying.

In order to be cured, all the cancer cells have to be dead.* In other words, there can be no rogue cancers cells still alive and hiding somewhere in the body. For a colon cancer patient who might have had surgery and chemotherapy, this means no cells hiding in the colon or any of the other organs, like the liver or lungs.

The problem is that for the vast majority of cancers, when treatment is finished, we can't be sure that there are no rogue cells. Our scanners cannot detect small clumps of only a few cancer cells. We can detect those clumps only once they grow into a tumor that is at least a few millimeters in size. By the time tumors are detectable by our scans, they usually contain at least millions—if not billions—of cells.

We could scan a patient with lung cancer immediately after treatment and not see any spots of cancer anywhere in the body, but that doesn't mean that there aren't any cancer cells hiding somewhere. A clear scan just means there are no spots of cancer more than a few millimeters in size. The patient could still develop spots of lung cancer in the liver a few years later, cells that hid in the liver before the original cancer was removed. Researchers are working on

---

* Emerging data suggests that in some patients who are cured, the cancer cells are not dead but just dormant, so they can't divide.

new techniques to find these spots sooner, but for now, we have no way to detect them when they are very small, and we have to wait some years after treatment to know that there are no spots of cancer hiding anywhere.

Some cancers do have blood markers that can alert us to whether a cancer has come back. This can be true for prostate cancer (using the *prostate-specific antigen*—or PSA—test), some colon cancers, thyroid cancer, and a few others. If these blood markers start to increase, doctors can go looking with scans to try to find where the cancer can be. However, just like with scans, the blood markers can still be normal even if there are a small number of cancer cells that could grow back later.

For cancers, the only way we know someone is cured is by the test of time. After a few years of close monitoring, if no spots of cancer are detected, it becomes less and less likely that any rogue cells are hiding. For many cancers, we set a threshold of five years. If nothing is detected by that point, then the patient is considered cured. Some cancers require monitoring even longer. "Cure" is a diagnosis that we can make only in hindsight, after enough time has passed and nothing has come back.

More Lingo: Our Mission Is Remission

Let's review some of the words that are used to describe whether the treatment has been successful or not.

For some patients, the goal of treatment is to "cure" the cancer. Curing the cancer means that it is gone and will never come back. The patient lives out her normal life expectancy, and the cancer will not end her life early. When the goal is to cure, we say that the treatment has a "curative intent," or we call it "radical" treatment.

Some cancers cannot be cured. If the goal of treatment is not for cure, but to either slow down the growth of the cancer, improve quality of life, or extend survival, then we call the treatment "palliative." The word "terminal" signifies a cancer that cannot be cured and is expected to be fatal.

So what does it mean when a cancer is in "remission"? Remission means that the cancer has gotten smaller, almost always because of a treatment that has helped. It doesn't necessarily mean that the cancer has gone away completely. If some or all of the tumors are still visible but smaller, then it's "partial remission." If all the tumors have disappeared from the scans, then we use the words "complete remission," meaning that there is no sign of any cancer. After several years in complete remission, we often say a patient is "cured."

What about being "cancer-free"? This can be a confusing term that is used loosely. We really only know that someone is "cancer-free" when several years have passed after treatment and he is considered cured. The situation becomes muddled because some people use the term "cancer-free" to mean "complete remission," meaning that the scans do not show any spots of cancer after treatment. This is not truly "cancer-free," because we can't be sure that there are no cancer cells still lingering until the patient passes the test of time.

Wrap-up and Key Points

This chapter is an overview of the basics about cancer. We've learned that:

- Cancer occurs when normal cells become mutated and develop the ability to keep dividing, invade normal tissues, and spread, among other traits.

- Cancer cells can cause problems, usually by damaging the tissue where they arise or damaging other organs after they have metastasized.

- Doctors will usually do a biopsy to determine the type of cancer, and they will determine the stage by looking for cancer in other parts of the body.

- The three main treatments for cancer are surgery, radiation, and systemic therapies.

- Doctors know that a patient is cured only after several years pass following treatment without the cancer coming back.

You can learn more about your specific cancer type (whether it's lung, breast, colon, prostate, or any other cancer) using the resources discussed later in this book. The more you know about your individual type of cancer, the better equipped you will be for your mission to take control of your situation and get the best-quality care. This mission starts with your first interaction with your cancer specialist: the consultation, which we discuss next.

Resources

Learning More About Cancer

To learn more about the cancer basics, see the "Cancer Basics" sections of the American Cancer Society website (http://www.cancer.org/cancer/cancerbasics/) and the Cancer.Net website (http://www.cancer.net/navigating-cancer-care/cancer-basics).

Online Medical Dictionaries

The National Cancer Institute provides a dictionary specific to cancer at http://www.cancer.gov/publications/dictionaries/cancer-terms. If there is a word that you can't find there, check the more general medical dictionary provided by MedlinePlus at https://medlineplus.gov/mplusdictionary.html.

Understanding
Your Situation

CHAPTER 3

Where It All Starts:
Your First Consultation

Your cancer treatment journey will usually start with a visit to a cancer specialist. This specialist might be a surgeon, a medical oncologist (who, as a reminder, is a doctor who prescribes systemic therapy), or a radiation oncologist (a doctor who prescribes radiation therapy).

This *consultation*—your first meeting with the specialist—is important because it sets the stage for all the tests or treatments that follow. At this consultation, you and the doctor will review the details of your overall health, your symptoms, and your test results. The doctor will usually do a physical exam. The consultation ends with a discussion of the overall situation and a plan for the next steps. The doctor might make a recommendation for treatment (such as having surgery, radiation, chemotherapy, or a combination), or the doctor might present you with a few different options for you to choose from. In some cases, more steps might be needed before a treatment plan is made—either additional tests or scans, or opinions from other doctors.

Going into your consultation, you should have two main goals:

1. To make sure that your doctor has all of the necessary information about you, including your personal goals and values

2. To make sure that you have all of the necessary information to make a treatment decision

To help you achieve these two goals, this chapter will walk you through a typical consultation visit. You will learn what to expect from the visit and how to make the most of this meeting with your doctor. First, we will start with ways to best prepare for the visit itself.

Preparing for Your Consultation

Your doctor can make good recommendations only if he or she knows your full medical background. If you have already assembled all your medical documents, bring them with you. Your doctor will want to know all your previous medical problems, so make a list of these. This list should include things like high blood pressure, diabetes, or a previous heart attack. If you've had cancer in the past, write down as many details as you remember, including how it was treated. If you've had previous chemotherapy or radiation, it can make a big difference in terms of treatment options.

You should also have a list of all your current medications and their doses, and you should bring the medications with you to the appointment in case anything is unclear. Update this list on a regular basis, bring it to all your appointments with all of your doctors, and inform your team of doctors of any changes. Make sure your doctors are aware of any over-the-counter or alternative medicines you are taking.

Bring a list of questions. This list will be built as you read the next few chapters. Also, bring a book or something else to occupy you, in case there is an unexpected wait. Although many of us try hard to run our clinics on schedule, even with the best intentions, we can sometimes be delayed by unexpected emergencies or by sensitive patient discussions that require more time than scheduled.

Take some time to reflect. A diagnosis of cancer is a time of tremendous change and anxiety. Taking stock of your overall goals and values is important to prepare you for some of the discussions that might occur during or after your consultation.

Bring a Sidekick

It's ideal to bring someone along with you to your consultation. A sidekick who knows you well, like a spouse or partner or close friend, can help you answer some of the doctor's questions. More important, your sidekick can act as a second set of ears to help you absorb information. This person can act as your secretary, writing down important information to make sure nothing is missed and freeing you up to just listen and ask questions. This person will also help you pass the time while waiting for the doctor and can provide emotional support. If you have a family member with a medical background or someone who has been through this situation before, consider this person for your sidekick.

Recording Your Consultation

Consultations sometimes involve complicated discussions. You will be telling your story and answering questions, and your doctor will be discussing your diagnosis, the results of your tests, options for treatment, and other important matters. Your doctor might use some words you don't understand. Your ability to absorb information will be hampered by the stressful nature of the situation. It is easy to get overloaded.

How much do cancer patients remember from their initial discussion with their doctors? Not very much. Doctors from Switzerland interviewed 71 lung cancer patients only a few days after they'd been told their diagnosis and the treatment recommendation.[9] The patients were asked whether they remembered the diagnosis (lung cancer), the recommended treatment (such as surgery), or the goals of treatment (curative or palliative). These are just the most basic pieces of information and barely scratch the surface of what you'll be learning in this book.

Patients did a good job of remembering the diagnosis and the recommended treatment—more than 80 percent got those answers right. But fewer than half of patients remembered the goals of treatment.

This finding is very concerning. Not understanding the goals of treatment has big implications. If patients don't know whether or not the treatment is intended to cure their cancer, how can they make good decisions about whether the treatment is worthwhile? How can they make plans for the future? If a patient thinks that a treatment is aimed at curing his cancer but it really isn't, he may choose treatments that are not right for him.

The stressful nature of the consultation is one of the reasons why patients can be left with a poor understanding of their situation. But some of the blame lies with physicians. Sometimes we skirt around sensitive issues regarding prognosis, we use imprecise language to avoid upsetting patients, and we let medical jargon creep into our vocabulary. Perhaps we could do a better job of checking to see whether our patients understand the message that we are delivering.

In light of the difficulty of remembering everything that is discussed, it's important to keep a record at your consultation, either by writing everything down or by audiotaping the discussion. If you choose to go with the pen-and-paper method, it's best to have your sidekick do the writing, and don't be afraid to ask your doctor to pause or repeat something to make sure all the important details get written down.

It's often easier to bring an audio recorder to your consultation. Nowadays, most people just use their smartphones. Studies show that most patients find audio recordings of their consultations to be helpful, and using them can increase patient satisfaction.[10] A recording can also let family members and friends who cannot attend the consultation listen afterward.

If you want to audio-record, just ask your doctor for permission at the beginning of the visit. Tell her that you don't want to miss anything and that you'd like to record the conversation so you can listen again later. Most oncologists realize that this is an important tool for patients and are happy to oblige.

Don't worry that your doctor could be put off by your request. Most of us are accustomed to our conversations being recorded. Just tell your doctor: "It can be hard to remember medical discussions. Is it okay if I record our conversation?"

The Consultation Visit

The consultation visit is usually broken into three parts:

1. The history: a question-and-answer period reviewing important medical details and symptoms

2. The physical examination: the doctor looks at, listens to, or *palpates* (feels) the relevant areas of the body

3. The discussion: where the situation is summarized and decisions are made

After the visit, your doctor will write or dictate a *consultation note*. This report covers all the important details of your medical situation and will be placed in your medical file. This will be one of the important documents that you obtain when you get a copy of your medical records, a process that we will discuss in the next chapter. As we go through this chapter and discuss the different parts of the visit, I will give you an example of the relevant parts of a consultation note. This will help you to follow along with your own report. The sample consultation note we will use here is for a patient with lung cancer, but consultation notes are usually very similar regardless of the type of cancer we are dealing with. After each section of the sample consultation note, I will provide an explanation to help decipher it.

Figuring Out Who's Who

Sometimes all the elements that make up a consultation (the history, the physical exam, and the discussion) will be done directly by your doctor. More commonly, though, some questions are asked using a questionnaire—to ensure nothing is missed—or by another team member.

Some oncologists seem to have an army of team members working with them, particularly if they work at a teaching hospital. These team members might carry out parts of the consultation and then report to the doctor in charge. These people can be fully trained team members, such as nurses, nurse-practitioners, physician assistants, and "learners," including doctors-in-training at various stages of their education or nursing students. It is easy to get confused as to who does what, and introductions might happen quickly, leaving you without an idea of who you're talking to.

Confusing things further, doctors-in-training can have different titles with unclear meanings, such as clerks, interns, residents, registrars, or fellows. If you're not sure of someone's role, just ask.

Part I: The History

Your Current Symptoms

The *history* is the retelling of your story. Your doctor needs to know about your current symptoms, the tests you've had done, your other medical issues, and other important facts about your life and health.

The first part of the history is often titled the "History of Present Illness." This is the set of events or symptoms that led you to seek medical attention. For example, a patient might go to his doctor because of a cough, which leads to a chest X-ray, some further scans, and ultimately, a diagnosis of lung cancer. Another patient may have detected a new breast lump while in the shower, which ultimately led to an ultrasound and biopsy.

The next step is generally known as the "Review of Systems." In this section, you will be asked a series of structured questions to make sure that no important symptoms are missed. In order to make sure nothing is omitted, we often ask about symptoms in a very systematic way, and many doctors just start with the top of the body and work their way downward. The Review of Systems might ask if you've had any headaches or any fevers, then move on to asking about any problems with vision, hearing, eating, or swallowing. Next, moving down the body, you might be asked about any problems relating to the chest area, such as problems with breathing, coughing, or chest pain, then questions about the abdomen, and so on. Eventually, all the important potential symptoms are covered, including symptoms that might be related to your heart, lungs, bowels, bladder, reproductive system, brain, and general symptoms like weight loss, fatigue, sweats, and chills. Doctors should also ask about your mood.

This section seems tedious but is extremely useful because it can provide important clues. If your doctor discovers that you've been having headaches or back pain, for example, it might lead to a search to check if the cancer has traveled to those areas. Symptoms that might seem unrelated to the cancer at hand could end up providing crucial information. Because this section is so detailed and methodical, it is often done using a questionnaire.

Your doctor might also ask about your *performance status*—your current level of day-to-day functioning. Your performance status is a measure of your present level of activity: Can you do all your usual activities, or are you limited in some ways? Are you up and about during the day, or spending most of your day in a chair or bed? Can you do basic self-care tasks, or do you need help from others? Patients with a good performance status are generally able to tolerate more aggressive treatments, if needed. If the performance status is poor (as in spending most of the day in bed), less aggressive approaches are usually recommended.

In a consultation note, these first two parts of a history might read like this:

> Mr. Jones is a 69-year-old man who presents with a four-week history of cough, productive of yellow sputum streaked with blood, along with shortness of breath when climbing stairs and progressive fatigue. He was seen by his family doctor for the cough and started on a one-week course of antibiotics with no improvement. A chest X-ray showed an opacity in his right lower lobe, and a CT scan of the chest showed a mass in the right lower lobe measuring 4.3 cm in largest dimension, with a 1.5 cm enlarged hilar lymph node. A biopsy of this mass is pending.
>
> On review of systems, Mr. Jones also reports an unintentional 15-pound weight loss over the past three months. He denies any headaches, nausea or vomiting, or other sites of pain. He has no neurological symptoms or gastrointestinal symptoms, and the remainder of the Review of Systems is negative. Because of the shortness of breath, he currently spends most of his day sitting in a chair.

In this note, you see that the first few sentences tell about the symptoms that led to the diagnosis (the History of Present Illness), and then some of the test results are described. In some notes, the test results will be in a separate section (often titled "Investigations"). The second paragraph tells of the Review of Systems, and "the remainder is negative" means that nothing else informative was discovered.

Your Previous Medical Issues

Your doctor also needs complete information about your medical past. In this section of your history, your doctor will ask about your:

- Past medical history: any previous medical issues, surgeries, or procedures

- Current medications and their doses

- Allergies: to medications or to other things (like latex)

- Family history: who in your family has had cancer and at what ages

- Social history: this catchall category includes several important things, like smoking history, history of alcohol or drug use, previous employment, previous exposures to *carcinogens* (substances that cause cancer, such as asbestos), details of your current relationship and family, and financial or insurance issues

- Reproductive or sexual history, depending on your diagnosis: sexual history is most relevant for cancers that are related to sexually transmitted viruses, like cervical cancers that are caused by the human papillomavirus (HPV); the female reproductive history asks about age of first menstrual period, age of menopause, number of pregnancies, and use of hormone replacement, as these can be risk factors for some cancers, including breast cancer

The consultation note might read like this:

Past medical history: Remarkable for hypertension, type 2 diabetes, and a remote wrist fracture.

Medications: Hydrochlorothiazide 10 mg daily and metformin 500 mg twice daily.

Allergies: No known drug allergies.

Family history: His mother had breast cancer at age 70, and his father had type 2 diabetes. One brother had prostate cancer diagnosed at age 50.

Social history: Mr. Jones has a 30-pack-year history of smoking and quit 10 years ago. He drinks one serving of alcohol per day and denies any illicit drug use. He is married, with two teenage children living at home. He works as an electrician and has no previous occupational exposures to asbestos.

In this section of the note, we learn about Mr. Jones's previous medical issues, including hypertension (high blood pressure), diabetes, and an old ("remote") broken wrist. His medications and allergies are then listed, along with the elements of his family history and social history. A "30-pack-year history" of smoking means one pack per day for 30 years, or an equivalent amount, such as two packs per day for 15 years.

Part II: The Physical Exam

After the history is completed, a physical examination is usually done next. The physical examination involves looking at, listening to, and palpating (feeling) important areas of your body to provide more information about your diagnosis or any other medical issues. For this section of the consultation, you might be wearing a gown. Some people prefer to have their sidekick in the room with them; others prefer to be alone with the doctor. This is your choice. For examination of sensitive areas, if you didn't bring a sidekick but don't want to be alone during the examination, you can ask your doctor to bring a nurse into the room. Some doctors do this anyway.

Your doctor will usually examine you most thoroughly on your very first visit. On subsequent visits, the examination might be more targeted to the areas in question. Depending on the diagnosis, the examination could involve palpating for enlarged lymph nodes in your neck, armpits, or groin; looking into your mouth and ears; listening to your lungs and heart; and listening to and palpating your abdomen. Sometimes the doctor will test your strength, sensation, or reflexes. For some cancers, such as gynecological, prostate, or rectal cancers, an internal examination might be required.

The examination might also involve looking inside your body with an *endoscope,* a special kind of camera. When I see a patient with a cancer of the voice box, I pass an endoscope through one nostril to the back of the nose and down into the throat so I can see the voice box. Other times, the doctor will look into the bladder or colon with a similar device.

The consultation note for this section might read accordingly:

On physical exam, Mr. Jones looks well. His blood pressure is 125/80, heart rate 84, respiratory rate 16, and he is afebrile. There is no lymph-adenopathy detectable in the neck or axillae. Auscultation of the chest reveals decreased air entry in the right base, with no crackles or wheezes. Normal heart sounds are audible without extra sounds or murmurs. Abdomen is soft and nontender with no masses or enlarged organs palpable.

The physical examination section here starts with a list of vital signs (blood pressure, heart rate, breathing rate, and temperature; "afebrile" means no fever). The note then states there are no enlarged lymph nodes ("no lymphadenopathy") found in the neck or armpits. Listening to the chest ("auscultation") showed some reduced air entry in the lower part of the right lung. The heart and abdominal exams were normal.

As noted above, in some consultation notes, the physical exam section will be followed by a list of results from imaging and blood tests that have been completed thus far. We will discuss these test results in the next chapter.

Part III: The Discussion

The consultation then moves on to a discussion. Sometimes the discussion is very brief and straightforward, especially when more tests are needed before recommendations can be made. But if you are having a discussion of treatment options, this portion of your visit can be long and complicated, covering important issues and outlining the decisions to be made.

Each oncologist will take a slightly different approach to the discussion, but it often starts with an overview of the general situation. The doctor might say, "We are dealing with a breast cancer that appears to have spread to some of the lymph nodes in your armpit," and then go on to discuss the implications of this diagnosis and the treatment options.

Other doctors will take a different approach, letting the patient start the discussion. The doctor will ask you to summarize what you already know about the current situation. This is a safe approach that can avoid unwanted surprises for the patient and the doctor. By asking you to summarize what you've been told already, it allows the doctor to judge how much information you have already received and then tailor the discussion to your individual understanding.

Once your doctor is sure that you have a good understanding of the situation, the discussion moves to deciding on next steps. Sometimes more tests or opinions are needed. But eventually, either at this visit or later, you will need to make decisions about treatment. This is often where things go on autopilot: the doctor recommends a treatment (or you choose from one of a few options), and off you go. Treatment starts and you hope for the best.

Wrap-up and Key Points

In this chapter, we've reviewed the basic elements of your first consultation visit. You can prepare for the visit by making a list of the important parts of your medical history, along with a list of questions based on the other sections of this book. Consider bringing a sidekick with you and recording the conversation or taking notes. The consultation usually includes a comprehensive history, followed by a physical exam, and then moves to a discussion of next steps and treatment options.

Ideally, after the consultation visit or after any outstanding tests are done, all patients would be very well informed. They would have a full understanding of the treatment options, the goals of treatment, and the risks and benefits of all treatment options. But we know already that this is often not the case.

In your situation, rather than going on autopilot and hoping for the best, in the next chapters you will learn how to understand your situation and take control of your treatment.

CHAPTER 4

Deciphering Your
Medical Reports

The best way to get a full grasp of your medical situation is by obtaining your medical records and learning to understand them. Without a copy of all your reports and results, you won't be able to make sure that all the appropriate steps are being taken by your health care team, and you won't be in a position to judge whether the recommended treatment is really the best treatment for you.

Many of the scenarios in which patients have received inappropriate treatments could have been avoided if they had full access to their medical records. We learned earlier about patients treated by a doctor in Michigan even though they didn't have cancer; in that situation, patients obtaining a copy of their pathology report would have avoided that harm. I don't mean to imply that medical mistakes are in any way the fault of the patients. They are actually a fault of our medical culture. We don't empower patients, because we don't encourage them to access their medical records and truly understand their situation.

When patients don't have their records, they are relying completely on their health care team for all aspects of their care: to make sure all the correct tests are ordered, that all the results are received, and that any abnormalities are addressed. Some health care teams do an excellent job, and they have appropriate checks in place to make sure that the risk of a miss is low. But overlooking one report—or even one detail in one report—can have a big impact. Errors can occur when physicians don't read reports thoroughly and sometimes when physicians don't receive the report at all and don't go looking for it.

This chapter is focused on helping you to obtain and understand your medical records. I will start by providing some evidence of why it's important to obtain and understand your records, and then I will walk you through the process of getting organized and requesting your records. I then present a step-by-step road map to help you decipher your records.

Your medical records—and this chapter—will contain some technical lingo that might seem foreign at first. Don't be discouraged. In one of his high-profile books, Dr. Jerome Groopman, a professor of medicine at Harvard Medical School, quotes one of his mentors teaching him that "there is nothing in biology or medicine that, if explained in clear and simple language, cannot be understood by any layperson. It is not quantum physics."[11] After reading through this chapter and using the resources provided, your medical records should be understandable. They are not quantum physics either.

The Importance of Getting Your Records

Grace was a healthy lady in her thirties when she developed hearing loss in her right ear. She was referred to an ear, nose, and throat (ENT) specialist, who ordered a magnetic resonance imaging scan to investigate. The MRI showed a tumor growing on the nerve responsible for her hearing. That report was faxed to the ENT specialist, but he never acted on it.

The hearing loss got worse. Three years later, she was essentially deaf in that ear. She was sent back to the same specialist, who didn't mention the previous MRI result. He just ordered another one. The new MRI showed that the tumor, which was located on the nerve responsible for hearing, had grown—it was much larger and now more difficult to treat. Despite having surgery, she has been left with ongoing neurological problems as a result of both the enlarged tumor and the more extensive surgery required to treat it.[*]

If Grace had received a copy of her original MRI, she would have been able to make sure that the appropriate steps were taken the first time around.

But very few patients—only a small percentage—request copies of their medical records.[12] In my practice, even when my patients do ask for their records, it's mostly not for their own purposes, but to send them to insurance companies or employers for disability or insurance benefits. The patients who do ask for their records for their own purposes tend to be people who work in fields related to health care because they understand the importance of having them.

If patients knew the importance of asking for their records, these requests would be much more common. In studies in which patients have been asked whether or not they would like their records, they tend to be very enthusiastic, and the request rates are much higher. Patients just need to be prompted to ask.

I also see this in my own practice. I've developed a habit of reviewing with my patients printed copies of their reports, pictures from their scans, or images from their radiation plan. Once patients see that the reports are easily available and not too difficult to understand, they often ask for copies.

---

[*]   You can read more about "Grace" at http://www.qualitycancertreatment.com/a02.

Improving Communication and Catching Errors

Providing access to medical records allows patients to catch errors and to note whether their records are complete. Studies show that allowing patients to access their medical records can improve doctor–patient communication and, in some cases, make patients feel more empowered.

Negative consequences of obtaining your medical records appear to be minimal, but it's important to be aware of the potential concerns. A small number of patients have been worried about a possible breach of confidentiality, in case their records were to get lost. We will discuss later how to keep your records secure. Some people worry that by giving patients their records, they will become more anxious. This doesn't appear to be true. In most studies in which doctors actually gave patients copies of medical records, it didn't lead to substantial anxiety.

The biggest downside of obtaining medical records is that it can be difficult for patients to understand them. In my practice, I find that all it takes is a little bit of extra explanation to give people a good grasp of what the records are telling us.

Start by Getting Organized

Before you delve into your medical records, you need to start keeping track of all your tests and medical visits. This will ensure that you don't miss any reports. The easiest way to do this is with a worksheet, and one is available for you in the Patient Toolkit.* You can either print out the worksheet and fill it in by hand or keep an electronic copy on your computer.

---

* You can find this at http://www.qualitycancertreatment.com/toolkit.html.

Your worksheet will be organized into five sections: visits to doctors, imaging tests, blood tests, pathology reports, and treatments. For each doctor's visit, list the date (whether it's in the past or the future), the name of the doctor you visited, the type of doctor, and whether you've obtained a copy of the report from that visit. You should also add any notes about that visit, such as recommendations made by the doctor. For imaging tests and blood tests, include a description of the findings.

How do you keep everything confidential? There are several strategies. One option is to go all electronic: start by using the worksheet on your computer. The worksheet can be password-protected and stored on an encrypted drive (see the Patient Toolkit video for how to do this).* When you receive paper documents from your chart, either type the results into the worksheet or scan the important documents as separate files, which you can also protect with a password. This will allow you to go paperless and destroy the paper copies. Make sure you create a backup copy of your files every so often. If you prefer to use paper instead, keep everything somewhere secure, consider getting a fireproof and waterproof container, and perhaps keep a backup copy of everything in case anything is lost.

Obtaining Your Records

In many countries, it's your legal right to get a copy of your medical records. In the United States, the Health Insurance Portability and Accountability Act (often referred to by its acronym HIPAA) requires medical records to be provided within a 30-day time limit.** The same right exists in Canada and many other developed countries.[13]

---

*　If confidentiality is a big issue for you, consult with an expert. No electronic security system is 100 percent secure.

**　To read about the US regulations on health records by state, go to http://www.qualitycancertreatment.com/a02.

Hospitals and doctors' offices have differing policies about exactly how you request a copy of your records and whether there is a cost. At many centers, you have to sign a request and pay a modest fee, but others allow you to view your records electronically for free.

If there is a fee, in some cases, there are legal limits to how much you can be charged, and patients who cannot pay cannot be denied copies of their medical records. Some centers also have financial assistance programs that may be able to help. Ask your doctor and the office staff how to get your records and whether the fee can be waived if the documents are for personal use.

There are also some shortcuts you can take. First, you don't need your whole medical record, just the parts that pertain to your diagnosis of cancer. Second, if you are seeing your doctor to discuss a test result, ask for a copy of the report after you've been told the results. Third, when you go to have scans or blood tests done, ask the labs if they can mail a copy of the results to your home address.

Don't worry that your doctor could be offended by your asking for your records. Most doctors are used to requests like these. Just explain that it will help your understanding of the situation.

A Road Map for Navigating Your Records

To navigate your medical records, we will divide the process into three steps:

1. *Checking the diagnosis.* What kind of cancer is it and where did it come from? This information usually comes from a biopsy.

2. *Determining the stage.* The stage of the cancer, as discussed earlier, tells us how big the cancer is and how it has spread.

3. *Considering individual factors.* Take into consideration factors that are unique to you, including your general health,

medical problems, and preferences, to decide which treatment would be preferred.

This is the same general approach that doctors take when classifying patients with cancer and deciding on treatment: they make a diagnosis, determine the stage of cancer, and then incorporate each patient's individual circumstances into the treatment plan. Once you have the same information yourself—the reports and records upon which they base their findings—you can do the same thing, checking what the standard recommendations are for your particular situation.

To facilitate this navigation process, real-life examples of medical records have been included at the end of this chapter, and you can also watch descriptive videos via the online Patient Toolkit.* The example we will use throughout the bulk of this chapter is for lung cancer, because it's the most common nonskin cancer worldwide, but you can see examples for the three other most common types of nonskin cancers (breast, colon, and prostate) in the end-of-chapter resources section as well, along with a more complete report for lung cancer.

Step 1: Checking the Diagnosis

What you need:

1. Pathology report

2. Consultation note

In chapter 2, we learned that doctors take a biopsy—removing a sample of the tumor—to send to a pathologist. The pathology report will tell you your diagnosis. Pathology reports are usually definitive in determining what type of cancer you have, but there can occasionally be some uncertainty, and the pathologist might not be able

---

* You can access these videos at http://www.qualitycancertreatment.com/toolkit.

to determine exactly what type of cancer it is. If that is the case, the report will say so, and it will often list the most likely types of cancer that it could be.

In some situations, you might have more than one pathology report. This can occur if more than one biopsy is done or if a biopsy is done first and then a surgery is done later as treatment. For a woman with breast cancer, for instance, a standard approach would be a biopsy to confirm the cancer, then surgical treatment with a lumpectomy and removal of some lymph nodes.

The pathology report from surgery is critically important, as it often determines whether more treatment is needed afterward. For the woman having the lumpectomy with removal of lymph nodes, if the pathology report describes only a small cancer from the breast and no lymph nodes contain cancer, the treatment options include radiation to the breast, hormone treatment, both together, or, in some cases, just observation. But if the pathology report shows a tumor with *positive margins*—coming to the edge of the specimen— and cancer in the lymph nodes, the treatment could involve more surgery, chemotherapy, and radiation to a much larger area.

You will find a detailed explanation of how to read your pathology report at the end of this chapter. You should also read your consultation note, because the doctor will usually describe the results of the pathology report there. This description should help you to understand the pathology report and its implications for treatment.

Step 2: Determining the Stage

What you need:

1. Consultation note

2. Results from imaging tests

3. Staging tables for your type of cancer

As we learned in chapter 2, the stage of the cancer describes how big the tumor is and how far it has spread. For most cancers, there are four stages—technically labeled the *overall stage group*—numbered I to IV.

The overall stage dictates the treatment options. In this section, you will learn to determine the stage of your tumor. For most cancers, the overall stage is based on three factors:

1. The size of the primary tumor (the original source of the cancer) and whether it has invaded any surrounding normal organs—this is the *tumor stage,* or T-stage

2. The number and/or size of lymph nodes that contain cancer—this is the *nodal stage,* or N-stage

3. Whether the cancer has spread to other organs in the body—this is the *metastasis stage,* or M-stage

As a whole, this is called the "T-N-M staging system." By combining the T-stage, N-stage, and M-stage, doctors assign the overall stage group (again, ranging from I to IV). You can do the same thing for your own situation.

The T-N-M system is provided by the American Joint Committee on Cancer, and it's updated every few years based on new information. A few cancers are not staged using the T-N-M system, and these include childhood cancers and cancers of the blood (such as lymphomas). For each type of cancer, whether it's breast cancer, lung cancer, colon cancer, or others, the staging details are different. You can look up the staging system for your type of cancer online.[*]

For illustration purposes, a simplified version of the staging system for lung cancer is shown in table 1. It's worth working through

---

[*] For a complete list of links to the staging systems for different types of cancers, go to http://www.qualitycancertreatment.com/a02.

this example even if you don't have lung cancer because it will help you to see how the staging process works.

Table 1. T-N-M Staging for Lung Cancer*

T-stage		N-stage		M-stage	
T1	Tumor ≤ 3 cm	N0	No lymph nodes involved with tumor	M0	No spread to other organs
T2	Tumor > 3 cm and ≤ 7 cm	N1	Tumor in lymph nodes at the root of the same lung (the *hilum*)	M1	Spread to other organs, such as the other lung, bones, brain, or liver
T3	Tumor > 7 cm or invading important structures like the chest wall	N2	Tumor in the lymph nodes in the middle of the chest (the *mediastinum*) but on the same side as the tumor		
T4	Tumor invading very important structures, like the heart, trachea, or esophagus	N3	Tumor in lymph nodes on the opposite side of the chest or above the collarbones		

---

*   This table is simplified and shouldn't be used to stage your actual cancer in real life.

Once you assign a T-, N-, and M-stage, you can then check which overall stage that corresponds to, per table 2.

Table 2. Overall Stage Groups for Lung Cancer

Overall Stage	Definition
Stage I	T1 or T2 tumors (≤ 5 cm), N0, and M0
Stage II	Tumors that are M0 and any of the following: T2N0 (> 5 cm) T3N0 T1N1 T2N1
Stage III	Tumors that are M0 and any of the following: T3N1 T4 N2 or N3
Stage IV	Any tumor that is M1

You can see how the stage of the cancer changes quickly as the N-stage and M-stage increase. Any patient who has cancer that has spread to even one lymph node is categorized as at N1 and at least at stage II. Any patient who has a lymph node categorized as N2 is at least at stage III.

Recall that for Mr. Jones, the lung cancer patient we met in chapter 3, the CT of his chest showed "a mass in the right lower lobe measuring 4.3 cm in largest dimension, with a 1.5 cm enlarged hilar lymph node." The 4.3 cm tumor makes it a T2 tumor, and the 1.5 cm enlarged lymph node is N1 nodal stage. Looking at the tables, T2N1 works out to an overall stage II (more specifically, it is stage IIA, as you would see in the full staging tables; some stages are subdivided with letters). With that information, Mr. Jones would be able to check which treatment options are most reasonable (more on that below).

The staging is usually quite easy once you have the tables. For a patient with a 2 cm tumor and no spread elsewhere, it would be T1N0M0, which is stage I. A patient with a more aggressive tumor invading the heart, with lymph nodes on the opposite side of the chest and a spot of cancer in the bones, would have a stage of T4N3M1, which is stage IV.

For some cancers, the staging system is very simple, whereas for others, it is more complex. Many doctors have to refresh their memory about staging systems by looking them up online. So you should do what doctors do: look at the staging tables to learn how your cancer is staged using the most up-to-date staging system.

Information Needed to Determine Your Stage

What information is used to determine the stage? Initially, we use information from examining the patient and from scans. This is the *clinical stage* of your cancer. During your consultation, your doctor will have examined you to look for cancer in different places. Read the consultation note to understand if anything abnormal was found, such as enlarged lymph nodes somewhere. Using the information from the physical exam and the imaging tests, you can determine your clinical stage.

After a cancer has been removed by surgery, if surgery is the treatment for that type of cancer, then we use the information from surgery to determine the stage. That information is found in the pathology report. Once we have that information from surgery, we've moved to the *pathologic stage.*

Accurate staging depends on having the correct testing done. We can't find cancer unless we look for it. Some cancers, particularly aggressive or advanced ones, require more extensive staging. For lung cancer staging, in addition to a CT scan of the chest, often a *positron emission tomography* (PET) scan and specific imaging of the brain are required. For other cancers, very few scans are needed. In the setting of low-risk prostate cancer, bone scans and CT scans are not recommended because the chances of finding any cancer on those scans are very low.

More scans are not necessarily better. Unnecessary scans can lead to delays in treatment, extra radiation exposure, and false-positive results. For patients with a low risk of cancer spread, the chance of a false-positive result on a scan can be higher than the chance of actually finding cancer spread. A false-positive result—a red herring—can be a big problem, as it can lead your doctor on a wild-goose chase; or, if it leads to unnecessary procedures (like a biopsy of an uncertain spot), they can carry a risk of complications.

Incorrect staging is a common problem. Studies of lung cancer patients show that recommended tests are often omitted.[14] For prostate cancer and breast cancer, overtesting is common.[15] In one study, more than two-thirds of women with early breast cancer received tests that would be considered unnecessary by current guidelines. One-third of all patients who received the unnecessary test then needed another test to clarify an indeterminate finding—but none of those tests showed any cancer.[16]

Later in this chapter, you are going to learn how to find out exactly which scans are needed for your type of cancer. First, we need to review the important types of scans, to give you an idea of what kind of information your doctors are looking for.

What Are All These Different Scans?

Most cancers are staged using a combination of only a few different types of scans: CT scans, PET scans, MRI scans, and/or bone scans. These are the workhorses of medical imaging. This section will describe these scans and show you some pictures to give you a better understanding of the information that doctors get from the scans.

The simplest imaging test of all is not a scan but just an X-ray. X-rays show us a two-dimensional picture, much like taking a photograph. Figure 1 shows us an X-ray of a patient's chest.

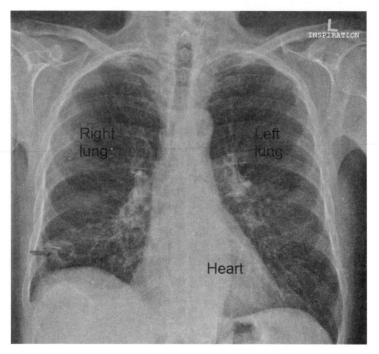

Figure 1. Chest X-ray. In an X-ray, bones are white and the lungs are black. The heart is also visible. The arrow points to a round white shadow corresponding to a cancer. It is much clearer on the CT scan below.

X-rays can be helpful, but they don't provide the same level of detail as three-dimensional scans, such as CTs, MRIs, and PET scans. Three-dimensional scans allow us to scroll through the patient, slice by slice, to see the tumor in much more detail.

A computed tomography scan uses X-rays to take a 3-D image of the body. On a CT scan, we are looking for the size of the tumor, any enlarged lymph nodes, and any other spots of cancer (such as in the bone or lungs). The CT scan in figure 2 is from the same patient as in figure 1.

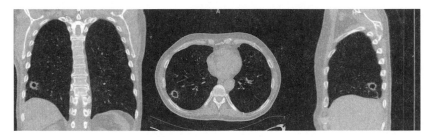

Figure 2. CT Scan. In the left-hand picture, you can see the tumor more clearly through the *coronal* view, which looks directly at the patient. The middle picture—the *axial* view—shows a sideways slice across the chest, where we are looking up from the bottom of the patient. The right-hand picture is a side, or *sagittal* view. Using the guidelines in the tables above, a doctor could diagnose this cancer as T1N0M0, which is stage I.

A magnetic resonance imaging scan doesn't use X-rays, but instead uses magnetic pulses to take a 3-D image. In figure 3, we see a CT and an MRI done on the same patient. Both scans cover the same area, but the information we get from each scan is different.

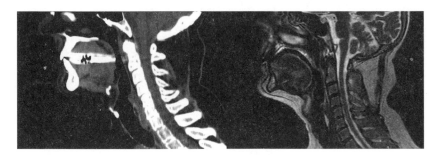

Figure 3. CT and MRI Scans. This is a patient with a normal CT scan and MRI scan of the neck. The CT is on the left, and the MRI is on the right. The CT is very good for looking at certain things, particularly bones, which show up as bright white. The MRI is better for soft tissues, such as the brain.

CT scans and MRIs give us anatomical information. They show us what is in the body, normal or not, but they don't generally show us which areas are active or growing. To get that kind of information, we use a positron emission tomography scan.

A PET scan uses a radioactive substance, often a special form of sugar (something similar to glucose) that can home in on tumor cells and cause them to light up in the images. The PET scan is often done at the same time as a CT scan because doing both together and overlaying them often gives better information.

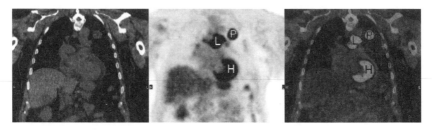

Figure 4. PET/CT Scan. The CT scan is on the left, the PET scan is in the middle, and the two images are fused together on the right. The areas that are dark on the PET scan (middle frame) and bright on the fused image (right-hand frame) are where there is sugar uptake. This includes the primary tumor (marked by P) and some lymph nodes (L). There is also some normal uptake of sugar in the heart (H). You can view a color version of this figure at http://qualitycancertreatment.com/links.

A bone scan also uses a special tracer that can target areas of bone that are damaged. An area of bone can light up on a bone scan because of a tumor there, but also because of noncancerous problems, such as arthritis or previous fractures.

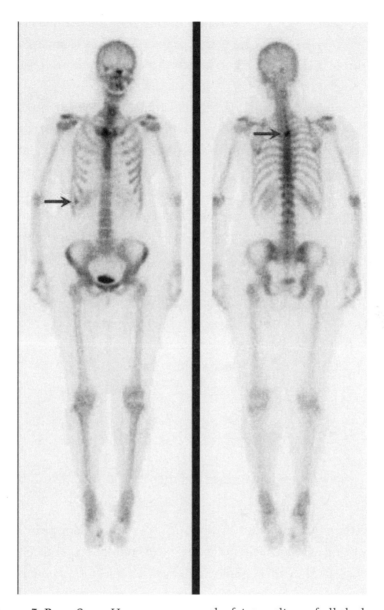

Figure 5. Bone Scan. Here you can see the faint outlines of all the bones, with a view from the front (left-hand frame) and the back (right-hand frame). Darker spots are where the tracer is deposited. There are two abnormal spots (marked by arrows), in the upper back and a rib. As you can see, it takes an expert eye to read these.

Detailed reports from several imaging tests are included in the samples provided at the end of this chapter. Use those samples as you read through your own reports, to better understand the results of your imaging tests.

Taking into account the findings from your consultation note, your imaging tests, and any surgery you might have had, and working through the examples, you should be able to determine the stage of your cancer.

Double-check this with the stage assigned by your doctors, and if there is a difference, ask why. Staging systems can be complex, both for doctors and patients.

If the level of detail of your medical records makes you uncomfortable, ask your doctor to explain what your stage is and which tests were used to determine the stage. Even this simple question can prompt a "second look" at your information by your doctor, to help ensure that nothing is being overlooked.

Step 3: Considering Individual Factors

What you need:

1. Medical history

2. Sometimes: blood tests or other special tests, like heart or lung function

Determining the stage of the cancer can narrow down the treatment options significantly. Sometimes, depending on the stage, there is one standard treatment approach. For example, for a women diagnosed with stage I breast cancer, the standard next step would almost always be surgery. Other times, there are several options. For many men with prostate cancer, the options include removing the prostate, internal radiation delivered by inserting seeds or catheters, external radiation delivered using a beam, or *active surveillance*, which means close observation. Choosing among these options comes down to individual factors, including how risky the surgery would be for an individual patient (this depends on the person's overall health) and the patient's preferences. Each option has its own risks and benefits. Different patients will make different choices, and different doctors will make different recommendations.

In this step, you take an inventory of your overall health, apart from your diagnosis of cancer. Make a list of your previous medical problems. Have you had major issues, like a heart attack, stroke, emphysema, or kidney failure? Or are the issues more minor, like high blood pressure or small surgeries? Have you lost weight without explanation? Double-check the medical history portion of your consultation note, where your doctor will have made a list of all the issues.

This inventory of your general health also includes assessing your performance status, which we discussed in chapter 3. Performance status is easy to assess. It is often measured on a scale of 0 to 4: a score of 0 means you are fully active; 1 indicates minor limitations (but you're usually still able to work); 2 means more major limitations (but you're still out of bed or a chair for more than half the day); 3 means you spend more than half the day in a chair or bed; and 4 means that you're bed-bound.* Performance status is important, because aggressive cancer treatments are usually appropriate only for patients with performance status 0, 1, or 2. When the performance status reaches 3, the benefits of treatment begin to be outweighed by the potential risks. Most studies of new cancer treatments don't test the treatments on patients with a performance status of 3 or 4. If you are spending most of the day in bed or in a chair, this fact needs to be carefully considered when coming up with a treatment plan.

---

* There are a few different scales for measuring performance status. The two major scales are the *ECOG score*, which runs from 0 to 4, and the *Karnofsky Performance Status* scale, which runs from 0 to 100.

After taking stock of your overall health, review any tests that your doctor has done to check your overall health. Depending on the situation, your doctor might have ordered blood tests or tests of your heart or lungs. We'll discuss below how to determine which special tests are required for your certain type of cancer.

You also need to consider your overall preferences about how aggressive you want to be. For most patients, the priority is to aim for cure, if possible. For others, the focus is not on extending life, but on preserving quality of life for as long as possible. In chapter 7, we will talk about weighing the risks and benefits of treatment, and at that point, your personal preferences will play a major role.

Once you have all this information about your health status, what do you do with it? You are not expected to determine how all your health problems impact your chances of success. There are doctors who specialize particularly in making that assessment, and it's not an easy thing to predict. But there are some tools you can use to help provide a good estimate. Because treatments are so variable in their potential side effects, there are very few general statements that can be made, but here are two specific parameters to consider:

1. Your performance status: If your score is not good (that is, if it's 3 or higher), generally the risks of more aggressive treatments outweigh the benefits.

2. Your age: If you are elderly, your tolerance for difficult treatments decreases and the risks of complications may increase.

There are also some evidence-based online calculators that you can use to give you a general estimate of the risks associated with some procedures, depending on your medical history.*

---

* For surgical risks, the American College of Surgeons National Surgical Quality Improvement Program provides a risk calculator at http://www.riskcalculator .facs.org/RiskCalculator. For chemotherapy risks in the elderly, see http://www .mycarg.org/Chemo_Toxicity_Calculator.

Here are some additional sample questions you might ask that take into account your individual situation:

- *Doctor, I had a heart attack this year. How does that change my chances of having a complication from treatment or my chances of success?*

- *I've lost a substantial amount of weight and spend most of my day resting in a chair. Does this influence your recommendation?*

Start Taking Control

You've now deciphered your medical records. You know your diagnosis and you know your stage.

Here are the questions you need to answer:

- Have the correct staging tests been done?

- Have the doctors assigned the right stage?

- Have the correct treatment recommendations been made?

Where do you find the answers to these questions? The National Comprehensive Cancer Network (NCCN) is often the best place to start. The network's website (http://www.nccn.org) is full of information specific to individual types of cancer, including breast, colon, prostate, lung, and several others. We will discuss guidelines in great detail later (in chapter 8), but for staging purposes, you can check the NCCN Guidelines for Patients® available on the organization's home page. There, for each cancer, the recommended tests for staging are described.*

---

* See chapter 8 if you need help accessing the NCCN patient guidelines. If your cancer is uncommon and not listed there, you can check the other resources in chapter 8 to find the required staging tests.

To pick back up with the sample case of Mr. Jones's T2N1 lung cancer, when we look at the NCCN guidelines, we see the following recommendations: CT scans of the chest and upper abdomen, blood tests, lung function tests, a PET/CT scan, a brain MRI, and a biopsy. For a man with prostate cancer, the recommendations tell you when a bone scan and an MRI or CT of the pelvis are needed.

As you read through the NCCN guidelines for your cancer, make a list of the recommended staging tests and check off those you've had done. If some are missing, discuss this with your doctors. And once all tests are complete, you can check to make sure that the doctors have assigned the correct stage.

Possible Errors to Look Out For

Here are some ways that mistakes are made:

1. *The pathology report is misread or inconclusive.* If this happens, treatment can proceed down the wrong path. Read your pathology report carefully.

2. *Proper staging tests are not done or unnecessary tests are ordered.* As we discussed above, under- or overtesting can lead to problems.

3. *Findings on a test are missed or ignored.* Read through all your imaging reports. Is there a finding somewhere that needs more explanation? This could include a lesion somewhere, such as in the lungs, liver, or bone, or an enlarged lymph node. If you are unsure of a finding, ask.

Wrap-up and Key Points

In this chapter, we've learned that obtaining your medical records can be useful to improve communication and to help catch errors. In many jurisdictions, it is your legal right to obtain copies of your medical records, although there may be a fee. It helps to start with getting organized, to help keep track of your previous and future records.

The road map to navigating your records takes the same approach that doctors often take in deciding on treatment options: check the diagnosis (mostly from the pathology report[s]), determine the stage (usually from imaging tests), and take into account individual patient factors, including medical issues and personal preferences.

Once you've deciphered your medical records and you understand your stage, it's time to think about treatments. But before we talk about specific treatments and which treatments might be best for you, we need to answer an important question in the next chapter: When doctors treat cancer, how do they know which treatment is best?

Resources

This section is intended to help you understand your medical reports. Generally, imaging reports are easiest to understand and pathology information is more complex. Use the online medical dictionaries (provided at the end of chapter 2) as needed.

I will start by describing how these reports are usually structured. Then we'll review sample reports for four different patient scenarios: breast, colon, prostate, and lung cancer. Together, these four cancers are responsible for about half of all cancer diagnoses overall. Even if you have a different type of cancer, these sections should be useful as you review your own documents.

How Reports Are Structured

Imaging Reports

Once a scan is completed, a radiologist looks at the images and creates a report. The reports are often structured into sections as follows (although there can be variation in the headings):

1. *Clinical Information:* the background history given to the radiologist by the other doctors

2. *Technique:* technical information about how the scan was done and if contrast agents were used

3. *Comparison:* statement about whether or not the scan was compared with older scans

4. *Findings:* a detailed description of what is seen in the scans

5. *Impression:* the overall summary of important points

Here is a sample of a normal imaging report, a CT of the head, with my notes in italics:

Clinical Information: 50-year-old male with lung cancer, R/O metastases.

The shorthand "R/O" means "rule out." The doctor who ordered the scan is asking the radiologist to look for, and hopefully rule out, metastases.

Technique: Pre- and post-contrast images were obtained.

Comparison: No prior scans available.

Findings: The basal cisterns are patent. The fourth and supratentorial ventricles are midline and undilated. The cerebellum and the cerebral parenchyma appear normal without any focal area of abnormal attenuation or pathologic enhancement. No surface collections or vault abnormality is seen.

Here, the radiologist is describing some of the key normal anatomy seen on the scan. Everything is normal.

Impression: Normal CT scan of the head. No signs of metastatic disease.

This is all the information you need: normal scan.

Pathology Reports

The pathology report will contain a detailed description of the specimen that is provided to the pathologist. These reports are also divided into sections, usually as follows:

1. *Clinical Information*: the background history given to the pathologist by the other doctors

2. *Gross Description*: the pathologist's description of the appearance of the sample that was submitted—how it looks to the naked eye and how it was cut up into pieces for analysis (this is the least important section for your purposes; there is rarely any critical information to be found here)

3. *Microscopic Description:* the pathologist's description of what is seen under the microscope

4. *Final Diagnosis:* a summary of the bottom line

Here is a typical pathology report for a biopsy of a lung cancer. Again, don't be discouraged by unfamiliar words. The language can be difficult to understand, but my notes in italics should help to decipher the report. You can go through your own reports with your doctor.

Clinical Information: Nodule right middle lobe found on CT. History of smoking. ? lung cancer.

This is the information provided to the pathologist. In this case, a nodule has been found in the middle lobe of the right lung. The patient has a history of smoking. The question mark before the words "lung cancer" is read as "query lung cancer," meaning the doctors are asking if this is cancer.

Gross Description:

A. LUNG BIOPSY: The specimen is received in formalin and labeled with the patient's information. It contains 2 tan cores of tissue measuring 0.6 and 1.2 cm in maximum dimension. It is submitted in toto in block A1.

Again, this is the least important section for your purposes. There is rarely any critical information to be found here because the "gross description" is what can be seen with the naked eye. The specimen consists of two cores of tissue and the measurements are given. "Submitted in toto" means the whole specimen was processed as a block of tissue, to be cut up and looked at under the microscope. They call the block "A1." In some cases, there will be more than one block, and they are named in order (A1, A2, A3, B1, B2, B3, and so on.)

Microscopic Description:

A. LUNG BIOPSY: Fragmented cores of lung parenchyma reveal a non–small cell carcinoma composed of large cuboidal to columnar cells with enlarged mildly pleomorphic nuclei, prominent nucleoli, and abundant amphophilic cytoplasm with frequent mucin vacuoles arranged in irregular glandular structures surrounded by inflamed elastotic stroma. A number of glands contain intraluminal mucin. The biopsy has also been reviewed by Dr. Smith, who confirms the diagnosis of malignancy.

This section describes what is seen under the microscope. In this case, the pathologist reports that in the lung tissue (called "lung parenchyma"), there is cancer ("carcinoma" means cancer). The pathologist then describes what the cells look like visually; these specific details may not be helpful to you personally, but you can look up the terms to decipher them fully if you like. In this case, the pathologist has also confirmed the diagnosis with another colleague, which is very reassuring and makes it unlikely that a mistake has been made.

Final Diagnosis: A. LUNG (RIGHT MIDDLE LOBE MASS), NEEDLE CORE BIOPSY:— ADENOCARCINOMA.

This sums it all up: it is a type of cancer called an "adenocarcinoma."

Your pathology report will tell you what type of cancer was found. Most cancers are called "carcinomas" (this one is called an "adenocarcinoma"), but cancers can also be called "sarcomas," "melanomas," and "lymphomas."

Pathology Reports from Surgical Specimens

Pathology reports from surgical specimens are usually much longer that reports from biopsies. With surgical specimens, the report

71

is often several pages long because the pathologist can provide a much more detailed description and analysis, as substantially more tissue is provided.

The sections of the pathology report from a surgical specimen are usually the same as outlined above (that is, a clinical description, gross description, microscopic description, and final diagnosis). But because they are so detailed, they often include a *synoptic report* or *synopsis*, which itself might be several pages long but just provides the most important highlights. These synoptic reports commonly also report the stage of the tumor, including the T-N-M stage if applicable. When the stage is based on a surgical specimen, doctors use the prefix "p" before the stage (such that a pathology report might report the stage as "pT2N1").

If you have a pathology report from a surgical specimen, the information you need most will almost always be in the concluding synopsis. If there is no synopsis, then the relevant information can be found in the "Microscopic Description" and "Final Diagnosis" sections. Here are some of the key features to look for in your report, as these can often influence which further treatments are needed:

- *How big is the tumor?* The size will be reported.

- *Does the tumor come right to the edge of the specimen?* The edge of the specimen is called the "margin." If the cancer is growing right to the margin, there is concern that cancer could be left behind. If cancer is at the margin, we use the term "positive margins." If it comes close, within a few millimeters, we say "close margins"; and if there is no cancer near the margins, we say "negative margins."

- *Does the tumor invade anything important?* The pathologist might comment on invasion into bone, into nerves (called "perineural invasion"), into blood vessels (called "vascular invasion"), or into lymph vessels (called "lymphatic invasion"). The latter two are often combined as "lymphovascular invasion."

- *Were any lymph nodes removed, and do they contain cancer?* If they do contain cancer, sometimes the pathologist will report whether the cancer is breaking out of the lymph nodes, called "extranodal extension."

- *What special tests were done on the tumor sample?* For example, breast cancers are checked for receptors for estrogen and progesterone, among others, as this tells doctors whether hormone treatments will work.

Sample Patient Scenarios

In this section, I provide case examples for four different scenarios: breast, colon, prostate, and lung cancer. Throughout the reports, I continue to provide translations in italics.

Each case takes you through the most common reports that are relevant for that type of cancer diagnosis. The documents included here are those that are recommended in the NCCN patient guidelines at the time of writing. I have not included pathology reports from surgical specimens, because of their length. They have the same structure as the biopsy reports, so you should have the background you need to understand yours, if you have one. If you need more help, see the "Finding More Help for Pathology or Radiology Reports" section later in this chapter.

Finally, radiologists and pathologists are often given guidance on how to structure their reports to be comprehensive and well organized. However, in real life, reports like those below are not necessarily structured accordingly. These sample reports are meant to reflect real-world reports that you might receive.

Example 1: Breast Cancer

The case presented here is a patient with stage I breast cancer. In this situation, the recommended investigations include bilateral mammograms, ultrasound if necessary, and optional breast MRI (among other investigations).

1. Mammogram and Ultrasound Report

Technique: Routine views were carried out of both breasts along with extended craniocaudal views bilaterally.

This tells us that both breasts were imaged, including a view aiming the X-rays from above to below (referred to as "craniocaudal").

Comparison: No previous studies available for comparison.

Findings: Both breasts show a substantial amount of dense symmetric fibroglandular tissue. A 1.5 cm soft tissue density is identified in the position of the palpable nodule in the upper outer aspect of the right breast. The nodule is poorly circumscribed with irregular margins. No other suspicious masses, pathologic microcalcifications, tissue distortion, or other signs of malignancy are identified.

The first sentence reports some dense fibroglandular tissue, which is benign. The key finding is an irregular-appearing abnormality that is 1.5 cm. It is at the location of the "palpable nodule," meaning a lump that can be felt with the fingers.

Ultrasound examination of the palpable nodule shows a fairly well-defined oval heterogeneous solid nodule measuring 1.8 x 1.1 cm. Color Doppler imaging shows some flow within the nodule. There are no enlarged nodes noted in the right axilla on ultrasound. Using ultrasound guidance, 4 core biopsies of the right breast nodule were obtained.

On ultrasound, nodule measures 1.8 cm. There is some flow on Doppler, meaning blood flow to the nodule. The lymph nodes appear normal, and four biopsies were taken.

Impression: Suspicious soft tissue density in the right breast. Successful biopsy under ultrasound guidance. BI-RADS 5.

This summarizes the findings above. The BI-RADS (Breast Imaging Reporting and Data System) score ranges from 1 to 6 and tells us how suspicious the radiologist is that there's a cancer.[*]

2. Pathology Report

Clinical Information: 1.8 x 1.1 cm solid nodule right breast.

Gross Description: RIGHT BREAST NODULE CORE BIOPSIES: The specimen, received in formalin in a container labeled with patient's information and "right breast," consists of 4 white-tan primarily fibrous and stringy tissue cores measuring 1.0, 1.0, 1.1, and 1.2 cm. Section code: A1–A2 specimen in toto.

As noted above, this describes the specimen: four cores of tissue each measuring about 1 cm.

Microscopic Description: RIGHT BREAST NODULE CORE BIOPSIES: Excellent core biopsies have been obtained which demonstrate extensive involvement by invasive ductal carcinoma (no special type) of estimated SBR grade 2/3. Selected slides have been reviewed by Dr. A, who concurs with this diagnosis.

The slides show invasive ductal carcinoma (meaning breast cancer) that is grade 2 out of 3. This pathologist has reviewed the slides with a second pathologist, Dr. A.

Final Diagnosis: A. RIGHT BREAST NODULE CORE BIOPSIES: — INVASIVE DUCTAL CARCINOMA (NO SPECIAL TYPE).

This summarizes the findings above. Often in breast cancer, the biopsies are stained for hormone receptors, but this was not done here and would instead be done on the surgical specimen when this woman undergoes surgery.

---

[*]   For more information about BI-RADS, go to http://breast-cancer.ca/bi-rads/.

3. Breast MRI Report

Indication: Right breast cancer.

This is the same as the "Clinical Information" section, just with a different title.

Technique: Breast MRI with and without contrast.

Findings: Breast parenchyma is dense. Mass in the right axillary tail measures 1.7 x 1.8 cm. No definite abnormal areas of enhancement in the left breast. No significant adenopathy.

The breast tissue (parenchyma) is dense. The radiologist sees only the known cancer in the right breast (near the armpit, in an area called the "axillary tail"). The left breast is normal, and there are no abnormal lymph nodes (no adenopathy).

Impression: Mass in the right axillary tail in keeping with known right breast malignancy. BI-RADS: 6.

The BI-RADS score is now higher, because the radiologist is certain there is cancer, since there's been a biopsy.

Example 2: Colon Cancer

NCCN-recommended tests for colon cancer include a colonoscopy and a CT scan of the chest, abdomen, and pelvis.

1. Colonoscopy Report

Indication: Abdominal pain and change in bowel habits.

These are the reasons for the procedure.

Procedure: Informed consent was obtained and the patient was brought to the Procedure Room. EKG, pulse oximetry, and blood pressure were monitored. Anesthesia was administered. In the left lateral decubitus position, rectal examination was performed, which was normal.

The patient provided consent and was hooked up to monitors. She was given some sedation and positioned on her left side. The rectum was examined.

The colonoscope was inserted into the rectum and carefully advanced. The descending and transverse colon appeared normal. In the ascending colon, an ulcerated mass was evident involving 75% of the circumference of the bowel. We were able to get past this mass and proceeded to the cecum and terminal ileum, which appeared normal. The scope was withdrawn back to the location of the mass, and multiple biopsies were taken and sent to pathology. The patient tolerated the procedure well.

This report describes that most of the bowel appeared normal until they arrived at an area called the "ascending colon," where a mass was found. Biopsies were taken.

Summary: Colonic mass, suspicious for carcinoma.

2. Biopsy Report

Clinical Information: Mass in ascending colon.

Gross Description: The specimen consists of 5 pieces of tissue, the largest measuring 0.6 x 0.3 x 0.2 cm. All tissue embedded, one cassette.

There were five pieces used for analysis.

Microscopic Description: Sections examined, see diagnosis.

Diagnosis: COLON, BIOPSIES: — INVASIVE ADENOCARCINOMA, MODERATELY DIFFERENTIATED.

This summarizes that the type of cancer is an adenocarcinoma. "Differentiated" refers to how normal the cells look: well-differentiated cells look the most like normal noncancerous cells, moderately differentiated cells appear abnormal, and poorly differentiated cells look very abnormal. These categories usually correspond to the grade of the cancer (see chapter 2).

3. CT of the Chest/Abdomen/Pelvis

Clinical History: For colon cancer staging.

Technique: A contrast-enhanced CT scan was performed through the chest, abdomen, and pelvis following the oral and rectal administration of GI (gastrointestinal) contrast material, and the IV injection of 100 mL of Isovue-370 (iopamidol).

This CT scan examined the chest, abdomen, and pelvis, and contrast was used.

Comparison: None available.

Findings:

1. CT CHEST: The mediastinum is unremarkable. In particular, there is no lymphadenopathy. The lungs are clear.

The mediastinum is the area between the lungs where enlarged lymph nodes might be found. This part of the scan was normal.

2. CT ABDOMEN/PELVIS: A small area of decreased attenuation adjacent to the fissure for the falciform ligament in the liver likely represents fatty infiltration. No further liver abnormality. The spleen and adrenal glands are unremarkable. A tiny calcification is present in the tail of the pancreas. Pancreas is otherwise normal in appearance. The kidneys are normal in appearance.

There are an assortment of benign findings that are unrelated to the cancer, including some fatty parts of the liver and a small calcium deposit in the pancreas.

There is a 4 cm mass in the ascending colon without obvious infiltration into surrounding tissues. Bowel is not dilated. No abnormal lymphadenopathy.

The mass seen on the colonoscopy measures 4 cm on this CT scan and doesn't seem to invade the surrounding tissues.

Mild degenerative changes are present in the spine.

These are age-related changes.

Conclusion: 4 cm mass in the ascending colon, consistent with the known colonic adenocarcinoma. No evidence for metastatic disease.

This summarizes the report.

Example 3: Prostate Cancer

For many prostate cancers, no imaging is recommended for staging. With higher-risk prostate cancers, such as a cancer that feels to be extending outside the prostate, recommendations include a bone scan (to look for cancer in the bones) and a CT or MRI scan of the pelvis (to look for cancer in the lymph nodes of the pelvis).

This case is that of a man whose PSA test (a blood test sometimes used to screen for prostate cancer) showed a rising prostate-specific antigen level in his blood. The PSA was very elevated at 21 ng/mL. When the doctor examined his prostate (using a digital rectal examination, or DRE), a lump was found on the right side of the prostate.

1. Biopsy Report

Clinical Information: PSA 21 ng/mL, rising. DRE: nodule at right base.

Specimen: A. Right base PZ x2(2). B. Right mid PZ x2(2). C. Right apex PZ x2(2). D. Left base PZ x2(2). E. Left mid PZ x2(2). F. Left apex PZ x2(2).

This describes the location of each biopsy. At each location (right base, mid, and apex, and left base, mid, and apex), two biopsies were taken from the peripheral zone (PZ) of the prostate, which is usually where cancers are found.

Gross Description:

A: The specimen consists of 2 cores of pale tan tissue, the largest measuring 1.3 cm and the smallest measuring 1.1 cm. All tissue embedded in one cassette.

A similar description is provided for samples B through F, so that information has been truncated here.

Microscopic Description: A–F: PROSTATE BIOPSIES SYNOPTIC REPORT

A: Prostate biopsy, right base PZ:

2 cores positive for prostatic adenocarcinoma, Gleason 4+4=8, involving 20% of each submitted core.

The two biopsies at the base of the right prostate both show cancer. In prostate cancer, the grade of the cancer is given in terms of the Gleason score, and a score of 8 means this is a high-grade cancer. All the rest of the biopsies (B to F below) are negative.

B: Prostate biopsy, right mid PZ:

negative for prostatic adenocarcinoma.

C: Prostate biopsy, right apex PZ:

negative for prostatic adenocarcinoma.

D: Prostate biopsy, left base PZ:

negative for prostatic adenocarcinoma.

E: Prostate biopsy, left mid PZ:

negative for prostatic adenocarcinoma.

F: Prostate biopsy, left apex PZ:

negative for prostatic adenocarcinoma.

Diagnosis: A–F: PROSTATE BIOPSIES: SEE SYNOPTIC REPORT ABOVE.

2. Bone Scan

Indication: Biopsy-proven high-risk prostate cancer. R/O metastases.

The doctor who ordered the scan is looking to rule out metastases in this patient with prostate cancer.

Comparison Study: None.

Technique: 692 MBq of technetium 99m MDP was injected and delayed images acquired. These were whole-body, anterior, and posterior images, as well as spot images of the head, cervical spine, thorax, and pelvis.

This is technical information, not overly helpful for your purposes.

Findings: There is no suspicious uptake identified at the skull and cervical spine region. Activity within the thoracic spine and lumbar spine is normal. Symmetric activity is seen at the shoulders. The ribs are unremarkable. There is no suspicious uptake seen within the pelvis. Activity within the lower extremities appeared within normal limits. The upper extremities are unremarkable. Soft tissue uptake appears unremarkable.

The doctor interpreting the scan is proceeding step-by-step down the body, describing the findings, and everything is normal.

Impression: No evidence of metastatic disease.

3. CT of the Pelvis

Indication: Biopsy-proven high-risk prostate cancer. R/O nodal metastases.

This scan is looking for metastases in the lymph nodes within the pelvis.

Comparison Study: January 2015.

Technique: Axial CT imaging of the pelvis was performed in 5 x 4 mm increments utilizing intravenous and oral contrast.

This describes the technical details of the scan and that a special dye (contrast) was administered.

Findings: Incidental note is made of relative asymmetry of the seminal vesicles, but this appearance is unchanged from January 2015 and is of unknown significance.

The seminal vesicles, which are glands attached to the prostate where cancer can spread, are not symmetric, meaning one is larger than the other. This hasn't changed from the previous scan, so the radiologist cannot be certain if this finding is due to cancer or just a normal finding in this patient.

The prostate gland is enlarged, but no evidence of abnormal intra-prostatic lesions.

The prostate is larger than usual, but on the CT, the radiologist doesn't see anything abnormal within the prostate.

There is no evidence of pathologically enlarged pelvic adenopathy. The bladder and visualized bowel loops are grossly unremarkable.

The lymph nodes, bladder, and bowels appear normal.

Impression: Enlarged prostate, but no convincing evidence of an intraprostatic lesion or extraglandular spread. No evidence of metastases.

Apart from the enlarged prostate, nothing else that is definitely abnormal was found.

Example 4: Lung Cancer

The case presented here is of a patient with non–small cell lung cancer, the most common type of lung cancer. For non–small cell lung cancer, it is recommended that patients undergo a CT scan of the chest and upper abdomen, among other tests, and depending on the results, often a PET/CT scan is recommended, along with imaging of the brain.

This case is more complex than the three above because it includes an abnormality found in one of the bones, which was ultimately biopsied to show metastatic cancer.

1. CT of the Thorax and Upper Abdomen

Clinical History: 65-year-old woman with lesion found in right chest on X-ray. Smoker. Query cancer.

The doctor ordering the scan provides the background information.

Technique: 3-D reformatted IV contrast-enhanced multiplanar CT of thorax and upper abdomen.

Technical details provided.

Findings: Spiculated nodule right upper lobe 1.7 cm. This is felt to be mixed ground-glass and solid. There is mild centrilobular emphysema. Small scar likely present within the lower lingula.

The radiologist describes a nodule with spiky ("spiculated") edges, which is often an appearance of lung cancers. The nodule appears to be partly a solid lump and partly "ground-glass," which means fuzzy-looking on the CT. There is some emphysema seen, consistent with the history of smoking. There is a small scar in an area of the left lung called the "lingula."

> No pleural effusion or pneumothorax identified. Major airways patent. Mild atherosclerotic calcification. Cardiac chambers unremarkable. Esophagus unremarkable. The chest wall soft tissues appear unremarkable. Lower neck structures unremarkable. No evidence of supraclavicular lymphadenopathy. No significant mediastinal or hilar lymphadenopathy by size criteria.

The radiologist runs through many of the normal organs, calling them "unremarkable," which means they appear normal. There are some changes suggesting coronary artery disease ("atherosclerotic" changes).

> Hypodense liver lesions likely represent cysts or hemangiomas. No splenomegaly. Pancreas unremarkable. No biliary tree dilation. Gallbladder grossly unremarkable. No evidence of adrenal gland nodule. No evidence of upper abdominal lymphadenopathy. Limited evaluation of the bowel is unremarkable. No free air or free fluid visualized.

These are the findings in the abdomen, with nothing to suggest cancer. There are some spots in the liver that appear to be benign, either cysts (fluid-filled structures) or blood vessels called "hemangiomas."

> Destructive lytic lesion in left T8 vertebral body. Remainder of bones appear unremarkable. Subcutaneous tissues and muscles appear unremarkable.

There is something destroying the bone in the vertebral body labeled T8. T8 means the "eighth thoracic vertebra," which is roughly one third of the way down the back.

Impression:

1. Right upper lobe lung lesion favored to represent primary lung cancer, likely along the adenocarcinoma spectrum.

Based on appearances, the spot in the lung is thought to be adenocarcinoma, which is a type of non–small cell lung cancer.

2. New T8 destructive lytic lesion. Considerations include metastasis and myeloma.

The radiologist suggests that the spot in the bone could be a metastasis or myeloma, a separate type of cancer.

2. PET/CT Scan

With a PET/CT scan, we are looking for *hypermetabolic areas*, or hot spots, which are areas where the radioactive tracer is accumulating. Hypermetabolic areas are suggestive of cancer, but they can also be seen with noncancerous things like infections.

Clinical History: Newly discovered right upper pulmonary nodule for further workup.

Technique: Approximately 1 hour after the injection of 463 MBq of F-18 FDG, a whole-body PET/CT was performed from skull base to the proximal thighs. The blood glucose at the time of injection was 5.3 mmol/L. CT scans were performed for attenuation correction and anatomic localization. Maximal SUV values were corrected for body weight.

This describes the radioactive substance that was injected. SUVs tell us how "hot" a spot is on the PET scan—higher numbers are hotter and often more suspicious.

Comparison: CT scan of the chest and abdomen dated May 2, 2015. MRI of the head dated May 12, 2015.

Findings:

HEAD AND NECK: Normal physiological uptake in the visualized parts of the brain. No enlarged or hypermetabolic cervical lymph nodes. Normal physiological uptake in the oral cavity is noted.

These areas are normal.

CHEST: Hypermetabolic irregular spiculated 1.6 x 1.4 cm right upper pulmonary nodule is noted with moderate FDG uptake and SUV max of 4.7. Scattered central lobular emphysematous changes are noted in the upper lobes bilaterally as well as in the right lower lobe. Hypermetabolic 1.2 x 0.8 cm right lower paratracheal lymph node is noted with moderate FDG uptake and SUV max of 3.8. No other enlarged or hypermetabolic lymph nodes. No pleural or pericardial effusion.

There are two spots of concern: the original tumor described on the CT scan above, along with a hot lymph node next to the trachea (called "paratracheal"). Both spots take up FDG, which is the tracer.

ABDOMEN/PELVIS: Normal physiological uptake in the examined abdominal and pelvic organs with no increased metabolic activity of the previously noted hypodense hepatic lesions. No enlarged or hypermetabolic abdominal or pelvic lymph nodes and no ascites.

This is normal. The report points out that the spots seen in the liver on the previous CT scan don't appear to be hot, suggesting they are not cancer.

MUSCULOSKELETAL SYSTEM: Hypermetabolic lytic destructive 8th thoracic vertebral body lesion is noted with intense FDG uptake and SUV max of 10.4.

The spot in the bone is very hot, further suggestive of cancer.

Impression: Solitary hypermetabolic right upper pulmonary nodule with hypermetabolic right lower paratracheal lymph node. Findings are in favor of a primary lung cancer with ipsilateral nodal metastasis.

Hypermetabolic destructive T8 vertebral lesion consistent with distant metastasis.

The appearance is most in keeping with a lung cancer with metastases in a lymph node and in the T8 vertebra. "Ipsilateral" means "on the same side of the body."

3. Bone Biopsy Report

The patient went on to have an MRI of the head (which was normal and is not reported on here because it is similar to the CT head report shown above), along with a biopsy of the abnormal spot in the bone.

Clinical Information: History of lung cancer and T8 lesion.

This is the summary of the history so far.

Gross Description: 8 brown-tan cores and multiple fragments; 3 cores are bony; the remainder are soft. Measurement(s): cores: 1.2 to 0.5 cm; fragments: 0.4 to 0.1 cm. Section code: (A1) 3 bony cores sent for light decal. (A2) 5 soft cores and remaining fragments—A2 is not decaled.

This describes the specimen and how it was processed, not overly important for our purposes.

Microscopic Description: Sections show ample core biopsies of dense fibrous connective tissue, trabecular bone, and trilineage hematopoietic marrow.

The specimens contain connective tissue, bone, and bone marrow. The term "trilineage hematopoietic" refers to the fact that the bone marrow is making normal blood cells.

The cores are infiltrated by cuboidal malignant cells arranged in sheets, nests, and rare tubules. They exhibit moderate variability in nuclear size and shape. They have moderate amounts of eosinophilic cytoplasm.

The key finding here is that the specimen is infiltrated by malignant cells. The pathologist describes what they look like under the microscope.

Immunohistochemistry: The malignant cells are positive for cytokeratin 7 and TTF1 (thyroid transcription factor). They are negative for cytokeratin 20, PSA, and PAP. EGFR (epidermal growth factor receptor) and ALK testing will be reported separately.

These are some special stains that were used that inform the diagnosis below.

Diagnosis: CORE BIOPSIES OF T8 VERTEBRAL BODY: — POSITIVE FOR MALIGNANCY, CONSISTENT WITH METASTATIC ADENOCARCINOMA, FAVOR LUNG PRIMARY.

The pathologist reports that there is cancer (adenocarcinoma) in the bone, which looks mostly like a cancer coming from the lung. This fits with the story above and provides a diagnosis of stage IV lung cancer. In some cases, doctors may then go on to also biopsy either the tumor or the lymph node in the chest.

Finding More Help for Pathology or Radiology Reports

Here are some helpful web pages that can help you better understand your reports (since the links to these pages are long, please go to http://www.qualitycancertreatment.com/a02 to see full URLs):

- College of American Pathologists
- Cancer.Net: "Reading a Pathology Report" section
- KevinMD.com: "An Insider Guide to Reading Your Radiology Report," by Dr. Rourke Stay

You should also review your reports with your doctors; they will be best equipped to answer the questions specific to your situation.

Understanding Blood Test Results

For each blood test, the laboratory will usually provide the test result along with the accepted range of normal values, so we can tell whether a result is within the normal range or not. For example, a common test for patients receiving chemotherapy is a measurement of *neutrophils,* a type of white blood cell. The laboratory report will state the measured value for the sample (for example, a neutrophil count of 4.0) and a range of normal values (such as 2.5–8.0). The result of 4.0 is within the normal range.

Each test will also have a unit of measurement. Neutrophils are measured in thousands of cells per cubic millimeter, so the reading of 4.0 really means that there are 4,000 cells in each cubic millimeter of blood. If you are looking at online resources, keep in mind that the units might vary in different countries.

The American Association for Clinical Chemistry hosts a useful website titled Lab Tests Online (https://labtestsonline.org) that explains laboratory reports in general (in the "Understanding Your Tests" section) and provides a searchable list of tests, with an explanation for each (see the "Tests" scrolling field on the right-hand side of the home page). The website also includes a searchable list of "Conditions/Diseases," including several types of cancers, with a review of some of the main laboratory tests for each one.

The American Cancer Society's "Understanding Your Lab Test Results" web page (also linked at http://www.qualitycancertreatment .com/a02) describes the most common types of blood tests used for cancer patients.

Evaluating Your Doctor's Recommendations

CHAPTER 5

How Doctors Decide
Which Treatment Is Best

In this chapter, we're going to discuss how doctors evaluate different treatments to decide which ones are best. As a cancer patient, this process is important to understand. Knowing how doctors evaluate treatments will help you to evaluate your own options.

I will first introduce you to *evidence-based medicine,* a process whereby doctors compare treatments to see which ones work best. We will then discuss how experts use evidence-based medicine to create guidelines for other doctors to follow. Guidelines help doctors keep up with the rapidly evolving scientific landscape and provide a framework for making decisions when taking care of patients with cancer. Later in this book, you'll learn how to access the guidelines that apply to your specific type of cancer.

Testing New Cancer Treatments

Let's imagine that we've invented a new anticancer drug designed to treat breast cancer. We want to test whether it is better than the currently available drugs for treating breast cancer.

We would first test this new drug to see if it can kill cancer cells grown in the lab. These cells might be growing in petri dishes or in animals, and we would expose the cells or animals to the drug to see if the cells die or if the tumor shrinks. If we can establish that a drug works in the lab, it might have promise for use in humans. But many substances that can kill cancer cells in the lab don't do the same when used in people, so this is not enough information to show that our new drug is helpful.

Once we establish that the drug works in the lab and is safe for animals, it is time to test it in humans. The first step is to establish safety, rather than seeing if the drug works, so we would give the drug in escalating doses to volunteers, to see if there are side effects. These tests are known as "phase I trials" and will be discussed further in chapter 12. But for the purposes of proving that our drug works, let's assume that we pass the safety hurdle and that we're therefore ready to compare our drug against the current drug treatments, which we will call "standard treatment."

In order to see if our new drug is better than standard chemotherapy, we need to create two groups of patients: one group that will receive the new drug (let's label them Group N, for "new") and one group that will receive standard chemotherapy (Group S, for "standard"). After treating all the women in both groups, we would wait a few years and see which group does better, either living longer or having the cancer in remission for a longer period of time. We compare the outcomes of Group N with the outcomes of Group S.

A critical feature of this comparison is that the two groups must be as similar as possible. If they aren't similar, the results will be biased. For example, if Group N is made up of women who have less aggressive cancers than the women in Group S, then the deck is already stacked in favor of the new drug. That wouldn't be fair and would give us an incorrect result from our trial.

The key question becomes: How do we create two groups of women who are similar enough to make the comparison fair? The simplest idea is to try to create two groups manually. For each woman who joins our study, we assign her to either Group N or Group S as we see fit. As new women join, we try to make the groups equal by keeping track of who is in each group already. For example, the first woman who enters the study could go into Group N, the second one into Group S, and then with subsequent women, we would assign them to one of the groups with the intention of trying to make the two groups as balanced as possible.

This approach won't work, for two major reasons. First, there are too many things to take into account when trying to balance the groups. Numerous factors affect a patient's survival, including her age, the stage and grade of her cancer, her performance status, and all of her other medical problems. Even with our best intentions, there would be too many factors to consider to actually balance out the two groups. The second major problem is that not everyone has the best intentions. A biased doctor—or a pharmaceutical company with a big financial stake in the outcome—could corrupt the process by assigning the healthiest patients to get the new drug, in essence stacking the deck.

The best way to create two equal groups is to assign patients to the groups at random. We do this by flipping a coin for each patient.* When the first patient enters the trial, a coin is flipped. If it comes up heads, then the patient goes into Group N, and if it's tails, she goes into Group S. For the next patient, the coin is flipped again, and the flips are repeated for each patient until the trial is full. Since we are randomly assigning women to the groups, this process will, on average, create two groups that are equal.

To see how this works, let's assume that there will be 30 patients with heart problems who enter our trial. It would be ideal to have equal numbers of these women in both groups (15 in Group N and 15

---

* In modern trials, computers are used instead of coins to randomly assign patients to groups, but the concept is the same. There is a good video available through the Cancer Research UK website explaining randomized trials at http://www .qualitycancertreatment.com/a03.

in Group S). The coin flip can achieve this. After flipping the coin for each patient, chances are that there will be about 15 patients with heart problems who flip heads and 15 who flip tails, so we should have an equal number in each group. Maybe there will be 13 or 14 in one arm and 16 or 17 in the other, but on average, it will be equal.

The same process applies to any other factor, not just heart problems. If you have 50 women who are smokers in your trial, after the coin flipping, you will likely have about 25 smokers who flipped heads and 25 who flipped tails. The beauty of this system is that this works even for factors we don't know about. If 30 women in our trial have undetected diabetes, 15 of those, on average, will be assigned to each group even if we are oblivious of their condition.

Clinical trials like these, where patients are assigned randomly to each arm, are called "randomized studies." Because randomized trials usually create two groups that are equal, they are the fairest way to compare two treatments. No other type of trial can even out the groups as well as randomization. That's why randomized clinical trials are considered the gold standard in medical evidence.

Randomized trials can sometimes yield surprising results, turning medicine on its head. Some treatments that seem very promising based on nonrandomized studies are later shown to be unhelpful, or even harmful, when tested using this gold-standard trial design.

Randomized trials are made even better when they make use of *blinding*, a principle whereby patients and physicians don't know who is getting the standard treatment and who is getting experimental treatment. In studies of new drugs, blinding is often done using a *placebo*, or dummy pill. For example, one group in a study might get the standard treatment plus a new drug, and the other group might get the standard treatment plus a placebo. Blinding removes biases— if you or your doctor know that you are getting a fancy new treatment, you might be more likely to think it is helping and more likely to say you are feeling better. For trials of radiation or surgery, blinding is much more difficult to do and is less commonly used, but it is still sometimes possible.

Doctors Don't Always Have Randomized Trials

Randomized trials are valuable, but they do have some limitations. The most obvious one is that they cannot be used to answer every question that doctors have. To illustrate this, one group of British researchers asked scientists to consider this scenario: you are flying in an airplane, there's been an emergency, and the plane is going to crash.[17] Your only chance of survival is to jump out of the plane. You have two options: put on a parachute before you jump or just jump without a parachute. The cheeky British authors point out that if you rely on randomized trials to guide you in this decision, you are out of luck. There is no randomized trial that proves that putting on the parachute will help. Their point is that not every question in life—or in medicine—can be answered with a randomized trial.

Like the parachute question, some medical questions also cannot be ethically studied in a randomized trial. To prove that smoking causes cancer, researchers could not ethically recruit volunteers and randomly assign half of them to start smoking.

In addition to ethical concerns for some questions, there are other reasons why randomized trials sometimes can't be done: sometimes the cancer is too rare, or the scenario is too uncommon, to have enough patients to run a study. Doctors try to overcome this issue by teaming up in large groups, sometimes with hundreds of cancer hospitals participating in a study in order to get enough patients. Other times, the cost and complexity of carrying out a randomized trial are too high. A randomized trial can cost millions of dollars to run.[18] It requires large numbers of staff to collect data, and it can take years, sometimes decades, to complete. It also takes very motivated doctors who will put years of work—sometimes all unpaid—into conducting a trial. Trying to lead a randomized trial on top of all their other commitments is difficult.

And even when a randomized study is started, sometimes patients or physicians do not want to participate. They might not like the idea of joining new studies, since they often entail extra visits or tests. Some patients don't like the idea of having their treatment decided by chance. Sometimes doctors have a strong feeling that one treatment is better than another and don't want their patients to participate.

One example of this unwillingness to participate comes from the treatment of prostate cancer. As we discussed in earlier chapters, there are several good options for treatment of early prostate cancer, including surgery as one option and *brachytherapy* (internal radiation) as another. Nonrandomized studies suggest that both treatments have good outcomes, and a randomized trial was clearly needed. But when doctors launched a randomized trial in North America to compare the two, most patients were not interested in having their treatment choice decided by a coin flip. Understandably, they preferred to choose which treatment they received, and as a result, the study never recruited enough patients.[19]

Because of all these barriers to carrying out randomized trials, in many situations, doctors just don't have data from randomized trials available to compare two different treatment options. This is an unavoidable part of medicine, and so doctors rely on other types of evidence to try to answer questions when randomized trials can't be done.

Doctors as Detectives

When randomized studies are not possible or haven't been done, doctors use other types of studies to give them information. Although studies that are not randomized can have limitations and biases, they can be better than having no data at all. For example, I could report the results of my lung cancer patients who were treated with a new treatment, Treatment X, compared with patients who were treated with an old treatment, Treatment Y. Other doctors will realize that this type of study is at risk of being biased because there could be some big differences between the patients in the two groups. To make my study better, I could use sophisticated statistical techniques to try to make the groups as comparable as possible and to try to remove the influence of extraneous factors. Nonrandomized studies are considered less useful than randomized studies, so doctors take this information with a grain of salt. However, as just pointed out, this information can be better than no information at all.

Without data from randomized trials, doctors also look for important clues as to a drug's effectiveness, including a biological explanation for why the drug might work and a dose-response relationship, meaning that more drug has more effect than less drug does, suggesting that the drug might be doing something. This is how we proved that smoking causes cancer. Just as detectives can still solve a mystery without a smoking gun, doctors can often still make good decisions without randomized trials.

This whole process—using different types of studies to make medical decisions, keeping in mind the limitations of each study—comprises *evidence-based medicine*. Evidence-based medicine integrates the data from research, clinical expertise, and patient values to make decisions about treatment. To practice evidence-based medicine, doctors have to be detectives, gathering evidence to make a decision.*

---

*   You can read more about evidence-based medicine at http://www.qualitycancer
        treatment.com/a03.

Evidence-based medicine is easy when all the studies produce the same result. But that is sometimes not the case. Disagreements can arise when not all studies agree or if some studies have weaknesses or possible biases.

Imagine two detectives at a crime scene. A weapon is found with fingerprints and DNA evidence on it. Eyewitnesses identify the criminal as the same person whose fingerprints and DNA were found on the weapon. This would be a slam dunk. Any two detectives would reach the same conclusion about who committed the crime. This would be analogous to having a good randomized trial (or, even better, several good randomized trials) showing that Treatment X is better than Treatment Y.

If there were no fingerprints or DNA evidence but two eyewitnesses both identified the same person, the case would not be as strong, but it would probably still be good enough for the detectives to agree and make the right decision. This might correspond to a situation in which a few well-designed nonrandomized studies all show that Treatment X is better than Treatment Y. But the detectives might be a bit less certain.

A worse scenario is one in which there are no fingerprints or DNA evidence and the eyewitnesses implicate different people. This would be analogous to a situation in which the available studies provide conflicting data. In this scenario, two detectives could come to different conclusions.

To summarize, in evidence-based medicine, if there are multiple randomized trials showing that Treatment X is better than Treatment Y, then it's very unlikely that two doctors will disagree on that point. But if the evidence is not as strong or is conflicting, then the doctors might each come to a different conclusion. And both conclusions might be completely reasonable.

Guidelines: Quick Summaries for Busy Doctors

One of the downsides of evidence-based medicine is that it is very difficult for doctors to keep up with all the new studies. Hundreds of cancer studies are published every day.* It is impossible to read them all.

To help oncologists keep up-to-date with the literature and enable them to correctly weigh the different treatment options, several institutions publish cancer treatment guidelines. These are usually authoritative, high-level institutions, operating at an international level (like the European Society for Medical Oncology), national-level institutions (like the National Comprehensive Cancer Network, mentioned in chapter 8), or lower-level but still high-profile organizations (like the BC [British Columbia] Cancer Agency, which we'll revisit later in this book).

To create guidelines, a group of experts is assembled. That group reviews all the research on a particular topic, assesses the strength of the evidence, and then makes recommendations. The process is repeated every few years to make sure the guidelines are up-to-date.

In some cases, the guidelines are very straightforward, recommending one treatment in a certain situation. But other times, when doctors don't know with certainty which treatment is best, the guidelines will give more than one option (such as surgery or radiation both being good treatment choices for certain cancers). Where uncertainty exists, the guidelines will say so. For the example of surgery versus brachytherapy for prostate cancer discussed above, wherein the randomized trial was not successful, we truthfully just

---

* To check this, I did a search to see how many cancer research papers were published on my birthday in 2015. The number was 300. Spending your birthday reading 300 articles doesn't sound like a lot of fun!

don't know which is better.* As a result, major guidelines don't recommend one treatment over the other.[20] Ideally, in this situation, patients would be made aware of the uncertainty and presented with all options. The problem is that this might not happen, as we will see in the next chapter.

Guidelines play an important role in ensuring quality of care, and we will look at them later, in chapter 8. They do have some limitations. Because every patient is a bit different, there may be some individual factors, like the factors discussed in chapter 4, that are not accounted for in the guidelines. Some doctors lament the fact that guidelines can relegate medicine to a cookie-cutter, one-size-fits-all approach. Furthermore, guidelines can become out-of-date and might not take into account certain things like the financial resources of the patient or the unavailability of some treatments in certain countries.

Even with these limitations, guidelines provide a very good starting point for decision making. We just need to keep in mind that treatment recommendations will sometimes need to deviate from what is recommended in the guidelines. When this happens, there should always be a good explanation as to why.

---

* It's possible that none of the major treatment options for low-risk prostate cancer is "better" than the others. As this book was being prepared for print, a randomized study was finally published comparing surgery, external radiation, and active monitoring for men with prostate cancer detected with PSA testing. After 10 years, in each of the three groups, only about 1 percent of men had died from prostate cancer. To read more, go to http://www.qualitycancertreatment.com /blog/changingtides.

Wrap-up and Key Points

The purpose of this chapter was to show you how doctors decide which treatments are best for their patients. In understanding the process and limitations of evidence-based medicine, you can appreciate why doctors sometimes provide differing opinions. One fundamental reason for differences in opinions is that sometimes the evidence is incomplete or imperfect. Imperfect evidence can lead to debates about optimal treatment approaches.

Guidelines help doctors by summarizing the scientific literature and making recommendations on how to stage and treat cancer patients. Where there are several valid options, treatment guidelines will reflect these uncertainties.

In the next chapter, we will discuss more contentious reasons why doctors sometimes provide differing opinions. We will explore why doctors might give biased information and how patients who receive skewed information from their doctors might end up choosing a treatment that is not really in their best interests.

CHAPTER 6

Is Your Doctor's Recommendation Best for You?

Patients put their trust in their doctors. And we as doctors are morally obligated—and in many countries legally obligated—to always put our patients' interests before our own.

Most of the people in my profession take this obligation very seriously. We strive to offer the best possible care, and we are very concerned for our patients' health and well-being. We think about our patients even when we're not at work. Many of us can recall being unable to sleep, even when tired after a long night shift, because we were still worrying about a sick patient.

But sometimes physicians falter in their obligation to patients, and their recommendations might not be in a patient's best interests. I'm not the first oncologist to write about this,* and I certainly won't be the last.

Why does this matter to you? As a patient with cancer, you might be navigating a situation where you receive different

---

* In chapter 1, I referred to the book *The Death of Cancer* by Dr. Vincent DeVita. DeVita writes that his colleagues were uneasy about his telling stories of physicians behaving badly, with one saying, "The public doesn't need to know these stories." Fortunately, DeVita disagreed.

recommendations from different doctors or where a doctor's recommendation might deviate from the guidelines we'll discuss in chapter 8. It is important to learn why doctors might disagree, how doctors can be biased, and how they can be influenced by external factors.

Why Doctors Disagree: Scientific Reasons

Disagreements among doctors can be beneficial. In many cases, when two doctors disagree, each doctor is suggesting a different course of action for treatment, and each can be considered by the patient.

This scenario occurs commonly, particularly in the setting of multidisciplinary team (MDT) meetings (which we will also discuss more thoroughly in chapter 8). At MDT meetings, which are also called "tumor boards," patient cases are discussed by the whole treatment team, including doctors from each of the different specialties (radiation oncologists, medical oncologists, surgical oncologists, and often radiologists and/or pathologists). It is common to hear many different opinions about treatment options before a decision is made.

As we learned in chapter 5, doctors often have good reasons to disagree—reasons that don't involve biases. Disagreement can occur because we interpret the results of studies differently, because we think that an individual patient's situation warrants an approach that differs from the conventional, or because of gaps in the scientific evidence.

How do we proceed in the case of two doctors providing differing opinions, both of which are evidence-based? The best approach is to provide the patient with all opinions and allow the patient to decide what suits him best.

Why Doctors Disagree: The Influence of Bias

Professional Biases

Let's consider a patient with stage I lung cancer—a small cancer that has not spread anywhere else in the body and should be curable (as shown in figure 2 in chapter 4). The debate over how this patient should be treated illustrates some of the biases inherent to medicine.

For more than 50 years, the standard treatment in this situation has been surgery, giving the best chance of cure. Radiation has been the second-choice treatment option, used mostly for patients who are too unwell to undergo surgery.

But the tides are shifting. A new type of precise radiation treatment has been developed: *stereotactic radiation.* The results have been very good, maybe as good as doing surgery, and with fewer side effects. Some doctors are now calling for stereotactic radiation to replace surgery as the treatment of choice. Ideally, we would now have randomized trials to compare these two options, but we don't. A few were tried, but not enough patients joined to allow for any conclusions.

Since we don't have randomized data, the truth is that we don't know for sure which of the two treatment options is better because we have incomplete evidence. If you took a poll of doctors, some might favor surgery, some might favor stereotactic radiation, and some might be undecided.

The problem is that doctors' beliefs are heavily dependent on what they do for a living. If you ask radiation doctors, 80 percent believe that surgery and radiation are equally effective in this situation. If you ask surgeons, the number is only 20 percent. And if you ask a neutral party (in this case, lung specialists who don't do surgery or radiation), the number is almost exactly in the middle: 49 percent.[21] Clearly, doctors are being swayed more by their profession than the scientific evidence. We see the same pattern in the treatment of men with early prostate cancer: the large majority of surgeons believe that surgery is better, but the large majority of radiation oncologists think that radiation and surgery are equally effective.[22]

The same biases also arise when you ask doctors about side effects of treatment. Radiation oncologists predict worse quality of life after surgery than surgeons do, and surgeons predict worse quality of life after radiation than radiation oncologists do.[23] It appears that doctors have a rosy view of the treatments that they themselves provide and a less rosy view of treatments provided by other specialties.

Because of these biases, the type of doctor that the patient meets can have a big impact on the type of treatment he gets. For men with early prostate cancer, a big determinant of treatment choice is the type of doctor the patient is seeing, whether it's a radiation doctor or a surgeon.[24] If you see a surgeon, you are more likely to have surgery, and if you see a radiation doctor, you are more likely to have radiation. The type of physician seen is even more strongly associated with the ultimate treatment choice than the patient's own preferences about side effects! This suggests that physician bias is spilling over into treatment decisions. We should be providing patient-centered care, where treatment is based on the beliefs and preferences of individual patients, but this data suggests that we are not.[25]

The bottom line is that specialists tend to favor whichever treatment they themselves provide. This bias, *specialty bias*, can be a major problem for patients. Patients rely on doctors to provide balanced information so that they can make an informed decision. If our opinion is skewed in favor of our own treatment—favoring our own specialty—can we really provide balanced information?

Compounding the issue is that once the bias sets in, doctors may be less willing to do studies to test their own treatments, for fear that they may lose out.

Dr. Tom Treasure is a British thoracic surgeon who has dedicated much of his career to undertaking rigorous assessments of surgery, including randomized trials, and challenging conventional beliefs. In discussing the debate about the optimal treatment of early lung cancer (the comparison of surgery and radiation we discussed above), he states that "in an era when evidence is expected for treatments, the fact that these interventions have still not been properly assessed is shameful."[26]

A big problem with these turf wars is that patients are caught in the middle, with no easy way to determine the best approach. "*Trust me, I'm your doctor* does not have the ring of truth," continues Treasure, "when different doctors claim to know what is best while consistently failing to encourage trials to put their beliefs to the test."

Financial Factors

Variations in the way that doctors are paid can create perverse incentives, rewarding behavior that shouldn't be encouraged. In some places, doctors are paid a salary, meaning they get paid the same amount regardless of the number of patients seen or treated. This is a good model to neutralize financial incentives, but it can lead to lower productivity. Doctors might be less willing to fit in an extra patient when they are on a salary, compared with when they are paid a fee for each patient seen. This latter model is the *fee-for-service* approach, meaning that more patients seen, and more patients treated, lead to more income. Fee-for-service models can be useful for rewarding extra effort: if a doctor stays late to see an extra patient, she is paid more. But these models can also encourage more treatments.

Reimbursement quirks can have unintended consequences and can change the way doctors practice. For many medical oncologists in the United States, the payment system for some types of chemotherapy can encourage the use of more expensive drugs, even when they are not necessarily better. In 2003, the US Congress enacted the Medicare Prescription Drug, Improvement, and Modernization Act, which stipulated that medical oncologists would be paid 106 percent of the cost of any drug they dispense.[27] This policy was meant to rein in higher profit margins that previously existed, but it had some unintended consequences.

Why 106 percent? The 100 percent was to cover the cost that the doctor paid to acquire the drug, and 6 percent was the fee for administering the drug. If a drug cost $100, the doctor would be reimbursed $106. The $6 would be expected to cover the doctor's overhead, with some left for take-home pay.

But this approach created an incentive to prescribe more expensive drugs. The 6 percent markup is a lot more money if a doctor prescribes a $10,000 drug (where 6 percent is $600) instead of a $100 drug (were 6 percent is $6). After the law was enacted, some studies suggested that prescription patterns changed.* Some doctors switched out less profitable drugs for more expensive ones.[28]

Other specialties also have similar problems. In the United States, radiation centers and radiation oncologists are often paid more for delivering longer courses of treatment. Reimbursement is higher for treating a patient with six weeks of radiation than with two weeks of radiation. Not surprisingly, when you compare patterns of practice around the world, this funding model is associated with longer radiation treatments—treatments that are not necessarily better but take a lot longer.[29] We'll return to this topic when we discuss radiation in chapter 10. For surgeons, the use of robotic

---

* To read a *Forbes* article about the impact of the 106 percent reimbursement system, go to http://www.qualitycancertreatment.com/a04.

surgery can be associated with higher reimbursement, yet in many cases, the benefits are questionable.[30]

These financial issues can certainly pose a problem. The good news is that many doctors can rise above these influences and are not affected. But it's important for you to be aware of the potential influence.

Pharmaceutical Companies

Medical-related industries, like pharmaceutical companies and medical device companies, can also exert an influence on physician behavior. We'll discuss this problem more in chapter 15. Suffice it to say that gifts or other items given to physicians, including food, honoraria, or consulting employment, can impact physician practice.* Ironically, physicians are likely to consider themselves immune from influence even if they receive gifts, but they are suspicious that other physicians are affected.[31] Even information provided by pharmaceutical companies can have a negative effect, even if no gifts are given. Physicians who have been exposed to information from pharmaceutical companies have been shown to write more frequent prescriptions, to use higher-cost medications, and to have lower-quality prescribing practices overall.[32]

Not Keeping Up with the Latest Developments

Cancer treatments change every year. It can be difficult to stay on top of all the latest developments, and keeping current requires a

---

* A riveting book on this topic is *The Truth About the Drug Companies* by Dr. Marcia Angell, a former editor of the prestigious *New England Journal of Medicine*. The book sheds light on some of the shady practices within medical-related industries and is worth a read if this topic interests you.

great deal of time and effort. Some centers and some doctors may not be able to keep up because of issues around time, motivation, cost, access to new treatments, or government/insurance approval of new treatments. It can also be difficult for doctors to move away from treatments that they have used for decades.

The difficulty in keeping up with new developments becomes clear in studies looking at the effect of physician experience (often measured as the number of years in practice) on performance. The stereotype is that patients prefer to have a more experienced physician, but the truth is that the opposite might be better. Across all specialties in medicine, the large majority of studies show that increasing physician experience is associated with *worsening* performance.[33] Specific to cancer doctors, increasing time in practice has been associated with less appropriate use of screening tests, a lower likelihood of recommending chemotherapy in situations with established benefit, a lower likelihood of adhering to guidelines, and less appropriate care overall.[34] Sometimes there is an initial improvement in performance during the first decade or so in practice, with a subsequent decline. These patterns likely represent the difficulty in keeping up with the rapid pace of change in modern medicine.

There is a difference between a doctor who is not keeping up with the latest developments and a doctor who is aware of the latest developments but doesn't feel that a new treatment is sufficiently proven to warrant its use. In the latter situation, the doctor should be able to explain his reasoning and feelings about the new treatment to justify this position.

Wrap-up and Key Points

In this chapter, we've learned that it's okay for doctors to disagree. Well-meaning, knowledgeable doctors might provide very different opinions in the same situation, and both opinions might be good options for their patient. But we've also learned that individual doctors are more likely to have a favorable view of the treatments they provide and a less favorable view of treatments provided by other types of doctors. We can also be influenced by financial factors and by industries in which profits depend on physician decisions. Sometimes doctors have trouble keeping up with the latest developments.

With your new understanding of how doctors evaluate evidence and why doctors might disagree, you can better sort through the different opinions you might receive from different doctors. In the next chapter, we are going to focus on how to use this information to decide what's best for you.

CHAPTER 7

Weighing Risks and Benefits

You now have the necessary background information about your diagnosis: you know about cancer, and more importantly, you know about your specific situation. It's time to focus on getting the best possible treatment.

The first step to getting top-notch care is making a good, informed decision about which treatment(s) to have. This involves, first, weighing the risks and benefits of each of your treatment options and, second, double-checking the treatment recommendations made by your doctors. In this chapter, we will focus on the first part: weighing the risks and benefits.

The process of understanding the risks and benefits is important to almost all cancer patients—in fact, in most situations, it is required by law as part of *informed consent,* a process we'll discuss below. Patients should understand the pros and cons of all possible treatments, along with the pros and cons of doing nothing, before making their choice. This chapter will provide you with tools to help you assess the risks and benefits of the treatment options available to you.

Curative vs. Palliative Treatments

The goal of treatment is usually described as being *curative* or *palliative.* Curative treatments are intended to get rid of the cancer.

If a curative treatment is successful, the patient will be cured and will be expected to live out his or her normal life expectancy. Curative treatments can also be called "curative-intent," "definitive," or "radical."

In other situations, the cancer cannot be cured, so the treatment is palliative. Palliative treatments are designed to slow down the cancer, to lengthen life, to improve any symptoms that might be occurring (like pain), and to delay the onset of those symptoms.

It is critically important to know if a treatment is intended to be curative or palliative, because this distinction plays a major role in decision making. If a treatment is intended to be curative, doctors will usually advise a more aggressive approach to maximize the chances of cure. The associated side effects, although undesirable, are outweighed by the potential benefits of treatment.

The situation is different when the goal is palliative. When survival time is limited, doctors and patients are more reluctant to compromise quality of life. From surveys of patients, we know that people with cancer are more likely to agree to an aggressive treatment if there is a chance of cure—even a small one—compared with when there is no chance of cure at all.[35] When you ask doctors to imagine themselves as patients with cancer, an interesting pattern emerges. Like patients, doctors are more likely to choose aggressive treatment as long as there is some chance of cure. But differences emerge between doctors and patients when the odds of cure are very low: doctors are less likely than patients to choose an aggressive treatment if cure is very unlikely.[36]

The overall message is that the goals of treatment are important because they determine the willingness of patients and doctors to accept side effects.[37] If there is no chance of cure, minimizing side effects takes on increased importance.

Without an understanding of the goals of treatment, patients cannot make well-informed decisions. As we learned earlier in this book, many patients aren't aware of the goals of treatment. A recent US study of patients with incurable colorectal cancer or lung cancer who were receiving palliative chemotherapy showed that a surprisingly large majority—69 percent of the lung cancer patients and 81 percent of the colorectal cancer patients—weren't aware that the treatment was not intended to cure the cancer.[38]

Many patients are frankly in the dark about the intent of their treatment. So when you are making a decision about treatment, ask your doctor if the goals are curative or palliative.

The Prognosis

The medical word used to describe the expected outcome of treatment is "prognosis." At one end of the spectrum, the prognosis for some cancers is very good, meaning that the patient has a very good chance of being cured. This is often the case with many early-stage cancers, including breast, prostate, and colon. At the other end of the spectrum, some cancers have a very bad prognosis, meaning that the chance of cure is low or that there is no chance of cure and the treatment is palliative in intent.

Not all patients want to know their prognosis, but most patients do.[39] For those who do, there is variability in how specific they want their doctors to be: some prefer to be given only a general idea of their prognosis (such as, "You will probably live a long time"), whereas others want numbers. And about 20–30 percent don't want to know at all.[40]

Knowing your prognosis can have several advantages. It can allow for more realistic decision making and more appropriate use of health care services. Patients often make better decisions when they are well informed and have realistic expectations.[41]

Whether to ask about your prognosis is a very personal decision. Overall, telling patients about their prognosis doesn't appear to be associated with increased sadness or anxiety, nor does it seem to worsen patient-physician relationships,[42] but of course every person is different. If you don't want to know your prognosis, that's okay. It's not critical, and you may not find it helpful.

Keep in mind that estimates of prognosis are just educated guesses. Survival numbers are just averages.* Some patients do better than average while others do worse. But if you want to know the average for people in your situation, ask your doctor: "What is my prognosis?" You can also check some of the resources in chapter 8 to get that information.

The Benefits of Treatment

For patients receiving curative-intent treatment, there might be other benefits besides having a chance of cure. Even if the cancer is not cured completely, survival can be lengthened or symptoms can be improved. These can be good reasons to have treatment, even if the chance of cure is low.

In situations where the treatment is palliative, doctors are looking for other benefits besides cure. In many situations, treatments such as chemotherapy can extend life for months, even years. For example, patients with incurable stage IV colon cancer treated without chemotherapy have a median survival of about 8 months. Using older chemotherapy drugs, as was done in the 1980s, lengthened that to about 12 months.[43] Now, with modern combinations of chemotherapy drugs, median survival is much longer.[44]

---

* Although I use the word "average" here, survival statistics are often described using the *median* survival time, not the average. The median survival is the time point at which half the patients have died and half are still alive. So if a theoretical group of 100 patients has a median survival of two years, it means that after two years, 50 will still be alive. For statistical purposes, using the median has some advantages over the mean, but in many cases, whether you use the mean or the median, the estimates may not be that different.

Ask your doctor about the potential benefits of treatment and how likely those benefits are. Is treatment intended to get rid of the cancer or slow it down? Is it intended to improve or prevent symptoms? What are the chances of achieving the goals?

Side Effects

Once you have an understanding of the potential benefits of treatment, it's important to understand the potential risks. Your doctors will tell you about possible side effects from treatment and the chances of each of those side effects happening to you. I've witnessed many doctors discussing the risks of treatment with patients. Often it's done properly, but sometimes it is not. Unfortunately, sometimes doctors gloss over the risks,[45] perhaps for fear of scaring the patient or to avoid uncomfortable discussions.

Keep in mind that everything in life comes with some amount of risk. This includes medical interventions. We have to be mindful not to overemphasize the rare events. As humans, we tend to worry about dreadful rare risks (like dying in airplane crashes), and we underemphasize common risks (like dying from slipping and falling).[46] While it's important for you to know about the rare serious risks of treatment, they have to be put into proper perspective by weighing them against the potential benefits.

We take risks only when there is a good chance of a benefit. If a surgery has a 1 percent risk of causing death but has a good chance of curing a cancer that would otherwise be fatal, most of us would feel that it's worth doing that surgery. When you think about rare risks, keep in mind that most cancers are eventually fatal if left untreated.

Usually your doctor will tell you the risks of treatment as part of her standard consent discussion before treatment. What do you do with the information about these potential risks? You can focus on two things:

1. Do these risks seem worthwhile, in light of the potential benefits? If the risks seem greater than the benefits, it can be cause for concern.

2. If you have a type of cancer for which there are multiple treatment options, you should compare the risks and benefits of each treatment in the context of your own preferences. One example of this is the use of surgery versus radiation for prostate cancer. If one option is more likely to cause problems with bladder control and the other more likely to cause rectal issues, you should decide which is more concerning to you. Different men would likely make different choices.

If your doctors don't discuss the risks of treatment in detail, ask them: "Can you tell me more about the risks associated with treatment, including common ones and serious ones, for each of the treatment options?"

Institution-Specific Risks

As we will see in the next few chapters, the risks and benefits of treatment often depend on who is doing the treatment. Specialized centers that treat larger numbers of patients tend to have lower risks of complications.

Patients and doctors can be lulled into a false sense of security based on the published data from high-performing institutions. If a specialized center has a low risk of complications, that finding doesn't necessarily apply to other centers. For example, for patients undergoing lung cancer surgery, a database of patients from a group of specialized US centers shows a mortality rate of 1.8 percent and a complication rate of 18 percent. But when researchers compared those numbers with data from across the United States as a whole, the results were not as good, with higher mortality rates and complication rates at nonspecialized centers.[47]

Doctors may not be aware of these differences, and they may be quoting the numbers from other centers, particularly if results from their own institution aren't available.

Ask your doctors for data specific to their practice or to their hospital: "What are the complication rates for patients treated in your practice or at this institution?"

The Goal Is Informed Consent

When agreeing to have treatment, you will be asked to provide *informed consent*. This is generally a legal requirement, except for a few situations, such as emergency treatments, treatment of minors, and people who are not mentally capable of giving consent. The specific requirements for informed consent vary in different states and countries. But in general, informed consent means that a patient agrees to proceed with a medical intervention with a full understanding of the risks and benefits. Informed consent also requires that the physician disclose the condition being treated (such as cancer), the details of the treatment, the possible alternatives (including nontreatment), and the risks and benefits of those alternatives.[48]

Consider a patient with low-risk prostate cancer who is choosing from among three options for treatment: surgery, radiation, or observation. These cancers can often be observed, but some patients prefer treatment. Proper informed consent means that the patient understands the diagnosis (prostate cancer) and that the treatment is aimed at curing that cancer (the expected benefits). He would understand that, for surgery, the potential side effects include more common issues like bleeding, pain, and infection, as well as rare but more serious issues like heart attack or death, along with the post-treatment possibilities of erectile dysfunction or urinary issues. He would have an understanding of how the side effects and potential benefits differ for radiation. And he would understand that without treatment, the cancer would be expected to grow, but that it might grow so slowly that it doesn't cause problems anytime soon and that treatment could be instituted later.*

Informed consent doesn't necessarily mean needing to know every last detail about treatment. It is important to have information about the potentially serious side effects, the potentially common side effects, and side effects that might be unique to you. For example, if you are a concert violinist, a risk of mild numbness of the fingers from chemotherapy might be very important to your quality of life, but perhaps less so for a singer.

In your situation, you should have enough information to truly provide informed consent for your treatment. If you have questions about any of these components of your care, ask your doctors before treatment starts.

Sometimes informed consent requires a period of reflection on your part to determine what is right for you. If you need extra time to think about the options, don't be afraid to ask, "When do I need to make a decision?" Your doctor can advise you whether it is in your best interests to make a decision sooner (within days, for example) or later (within weeks) depending on your situation. Rarely, treatment might need to commence immediately, and your doctor will advise you if this is the case. Even then, a few minutes alone with your side-kick to talk about the options can be valuable in helping you weigh the options without the pressure of the doctor in the room.

---

* This is a unique scenario. For many other cancers, observation is not a recommended option, as the chance of cure can be missed. If you want to read more about informed consent, there's a link to an excellent American Cancer Society resource at http://www.qualitycancertreatment.com/a05.

Wrap-up and Mini-checklist

This chapter has given you an overview of how to weigh the risks and benefits of treatment and the questions to ask in order to get all the information you need.

Starting in this section of the book, I will provide a mini-checklist at the end of each chapter that you can use to make sure you have covered most of the important issues discussed. These are the main elements of weighing the risks and benefits:

☐ I understand the goal of treatment (curative or palliative).

☐ If this is a curative-intent treatment, I understand the chances of cure (if I want to know that information).

☐ If this is a palliative-intent treatment, I understand my prognosis (if I want to know that information). Palliative-intent treatments are discussed in more detail in chapter 14.

☐ I know the potential benefits of each treatment option available to me.

☐ I know the risks of each treatment option available to me, including the results specific to the institution where I'm being treated.

☐ I have enough information to give informed consent for my treatment.

Before you make a final decision about treatment, we move to the next chapter to teach you how to double-check the treatment recommendations, how to get second opinions, and how to find tools to help you if you're having trouble making a decision.

CHAPTER 8

How to Get Free Second Opinions

It's important to get more than one opinion about your treatment. We've learned in previous chapters that patients can be swayed toward choosing their treatment based on the type of doctor they see first. Getting second opinions can prevent that.

When we talk about a second opinion, we often think about going to a second doctor for a formal visit in person. Although that can be important in some situations—and we will talk about that option in this chapter—there are other sources of second opinions, some of which are free.

This chapter will describe three different approaches to getting second opinions: getting more opinions from your own team, checking treatment guidelines, and getting formal second opinions. At the end of this chapter, I'll point you to some tools that are available if you are still having trouble deciding which treatment is right for you.

1. More Opinions from Your Team

Asking Your Doctors to Huddle Up

Football players often gather in a huddle to decide what they are going to do on the next play. Huddles allow the players to communicate and to make sure that everyone is on the same page. Cancer doctors often take the same approach.

Many cancer centers have special team huddles in which experts gather to discuss specific patient cases. These meetings are often attended by representatives from most of the cancer-related medical specialties. Attendees may include surgeons, medical oncologists, radiation oncologists, radiologists, and pathologists. They may also include nurses, pharmacists, dietitians, *speech-language pathologists* (who are speech and swallowing experts), *audiologists* (hearing experts), and other health professionals. Because there are so many disciplines involved, the meetings are often called "multidisciplinary team meetings," or MDT meetings, as mentioned in chapter 6. In some places, they are called "tumor boards" or "case conferences."

MDT meetings are designed around specific cancer types. For example, the MDT meeting in which breast cancer cases are discussed will be separate from the meeting in which lung cancers are discussed. The meetings are often held once a week or once every two weeks, depending on the center.

At each MDT meeting, patient cases are reviewed in detail to allow the group to provide opinions. A case discussion will start with a brief presentation of the patient's history and physical findings. In some cases, when there is a crucial physical finding to be seen, the patient might attend to be examined by the group in person. Next comes a review of all the imaging by the radiologist and a review of the biopsy or surgical specimens by the pathologist.

After all this information is presented, the group discusses treatment options and makes recommendations. Sometimes a strong recommendation is made for one particular treatment. Other times, the MDT affirms that a few good options are available and that the evidence is insufficient to strongly recommend one treatment over another.

MDT discussions can have a major impact on patient care. In 2016, an Australian group of researchers reviewed all the published studies looking at the impact of MDTs.[49] Most of those studies showed that more than 10 percent of patients discussed at MDT meetings had a change in management plans based on the MDT recommendations. In some studies, the number was much higher; in one, in fact, 52 percent of patients had some change in their management plan.

Why do so many patients have a change in their treatment recommendation? The Australian study explains some of the reasons. Sometimes changes in treatment occur because the MDT finds that some tests were not done. In one example for rectal cancer, the percentage of patients having the correct staging tests rose from 63 percent to 96 percent if the patient was discussed at an MDT meeting.[50] Correct staging can lead to different recommendations.

But even if the correct tests have already been done, MDTs can lead to different interpretations of those tests. The radiologist and pathologist at MDT meetings have two major advantages when they are providing their opinions. First, they specialize in the type of cancer that is being discussed. At breast MDT meetings, the radiologist will likely be an expert in breast MRIs. Second, they also have more clues to help them, because they get to hear the patient's story firsthand. If the surgeon felt something suspicious in one area of the patient's breast, then the radiologist can look more carefully in that area. These advantages allow the radiologist and pathologist to pick up things that were not seen the first time around.

The final major reason why treatment recommendations can change at MDT meetings is because more doctors are available to provide input. Basically, it's a roomful of second opinions, all provided at once.

There has never been a randomized trial for which some patients' cases are discussed at MDT meetings and others are not, to prove how beneficial it is. As a result, there is some controversy as to how much MDT meetings impact quality of care, and not all studies have found that MDT meetings improve quality.[51] This might reflect the fact that tumor boards are only one component of high-quality care; a center that is already very good at every aspect of cancer treatment might not see much more improvement with MDT meetings. Furthermore, MDT meetings occur at many cancer centers around the world, but practices vary. At some centers, all patients are discussed. At other centers, it might be only a minority (perhaps only the most complex cases) or none at all. At some centers, a radiologist or pathologist might not be present.

If you are like most patients, it makes sense to ask your doctor to discuss your case at an MDT meeting, as you might get a free second opinion about your options for treatment. Normally, your doctor will be happy to oblige.

Reviews of Your Pathology and Radiology Results

If you're unable to get your case discussed at an MDT meeting, or if the MDT meetings don't include pathologists or radiologists, those types of reviews can often be requested separately. A *pathology review* is when a second pathologist looks at the slides from your biopsy or surgery, and a *radiology review* is when a second radiologist has another look at your imaging.

Pathology errors are uncommon, but when they do occur, the effects can be large. One US study[52] of four institutions found pathology error rates ranging from as low as 1.8 percent at the best center to a high of 12 percent. And when errors occurred, they resulted in harm about 40 percent of the time.

In an extreme example, two women at one hospital underwent unnecessary mastectomies because of errors related to their pathology reports: the original biopsies were thought to contain cancer, but they didn't, and the mistake wasn't detected until after the mastectomies were done.[53] Pathology reviews in breast cancer result in changes in pathology reports in 20 percent of the cases, with a change in treatment recommendations in 6 percent of patients overall.[54]

Similar to the situation in pathology, radiology reviews can also be helpful. In a radiology review, a second radiologist reviews the imaging and issues another report. These second opinions can catch errors and lead to clinically important changes, with changes often reported in 10–20 percent of studies of radiology reviews.[55] The large majority of radiologists (more than 90 percent in one study) feel that these peer-review activities are worthwhile.[56]

This issue is so important that many institutions will do reviews as part of routine practice if you are referred there. If you have a biopsy somewhere else, they will obtain the specimen and have a second look at it before proceeding with surgery.[57] If you had imaging somewhere else, it will often be repeated so it can be read by their own radiologists.

It's worth asking your doctors if pathology and radiology reviews can be obtained in your case and if they would be worthwhile. These reviews are particularly useful when there are uncertainties regarding the pathology or imaging reports. If your case has been discussed at an MDT meeting, this might already be built in.

2. Consulting the Guidelines

In chapter 5, we learned about cancer treatment guidelines—recommendations for doctors on how to diagnose and treat cancer—and in chapter 4, we saw that there are also guidelines written for patients. The patient guidelines can provide a wealth of information and are relatively easy to follow. But they don't provide as much specific information as the physician resources do. So a good approach is to start with the patient guidelines first, and then move on to the physician guidelines. The downside is that the physician guidelines are more difficult to follow and will require some patience and perhaps an online medical dictionary (see the resources listed at the back of chapter 2).

Both the patient and the physician guidelines are usually freely available online. See the end of this chapter for guidance on where to find these guidelines and how to use them. There are also videos in the Patient Toolkit* that will talk you through the process. You can look up your specific stage of cancer, and the guidelines will provide you with the standard treatment options that can be considered.

3. Getting a Formal Second Opinion

Getting a formal second opinion involves meeting with a new doctor, and it usually includes a review of all your test results, including a pathology and radiology review. In some cases, the new doctor might want certain tests repeated or request some new ones.

A formal second opinion can lead to a change in diagnosis or recommended treatment. For cancer patients who get a second opinion, changes in diagnosis occur approximately 5 percent of the time, and changes in treatment recommendations occur about 20–40 percent of the time, although the numbers vary widely across studies.[58] Patients who obtain second opinions tend to find the process valuable—they report high levels of satisfaction and higher levels of confidence in their diagnosis and treatment choices.[59]

Seeking a formal second opinion has some potential downsides to consider. It might lead to a small delay in treatment, and it may

---

*   Available at http://www.qualitycancertreatment.com/toolkit.

involve some extra costs. If you are in an insurance-based system, as many people are in the United States and in some European countries, check with your insurance company to see what it will cover and if it will cover out-of-network doctors. You might be pleasantly surprised: many insurers are supportive of second opinions, and some even require a second opinion before cancer treatment begins. But if a second opinion comes at a cost that might be unaffordable to you, you can review the free online resources we discussed above first, before deciding whether there is enough uncertainty in the situation to require a formal second opinion.

There are no hard-and-fast guidelines as to when you should get a formal second opinion from another doctor. Some things to consider that might sway you toward a formal second opinion include:

- You want some extra peace of mind that everything is being done correctly.

- Some of your doctor's recommendations don't jibe with the guidelines, and you're not satisfied as to the explanation why.

- You don't get along with your doctor, or you have some doubts about his recommendations.

- Your doctor doesn't specialize in treating your cancer or doesn't have much experience with your type of cancer.

Although a second opinion is traditionally delivered in person, some cancer centers offer options for a virtual second opinion. Rather than going to see the doctor in person, you send in your medical records and/or imaging. They review those files only, without seeing you in person, and provide an opinion.

How do you choose a doctor for a second opinion? If you need to find a doctor for a second opinion, the resources listed at the end of this chapter provide some guidance.

If You Still Need Help Making a Decision

Sometimes treatment decisions are difficult to make, even if you are well informed about all the options. If you are still struggling to make a decision even after discussing your options with your doctors, here are some other actions you can take:

- Ask the other members of your health care team, including your family doctor, your oncology nurse, nurse-practitioner, or physician assistant, for their input.

- Seek the advice of other patients. You may already know someone who has been in your situation, or you can meet someone through a local patient support group or online. The Cancer Hope Network (http://www.cancerhopenet work.org) can match you up with a survivor of your type of cancer for you to talk to. The network's services are available to patients in the United States and Canada.

- Find a *decision aid*. Decision aids are tools that help patients make decisions. They provide information about the various treatment options and the risks and benefits of each. Decision aids have been built for many different situations, such as deciding on treatment in the setting of early breast or prostate cancer.*

- Meet with a cancer librarian. Many cancer centers have libraries staffed by cancer librarians. The librarian can help find answers to some of your questions and help you locate support groups and decision aids.

---

* A searchable list of decision aids is available at https://decisionaid.ohri.ca. You can enter a search topic (for instance, "breast cancer") to find what you are looking for.

Wrap-up and Mini-checklist

In this chapter, we've learned three major approaches to getting additional opinions on the treatment of your cancer. The first route is getting more opinions from your own treatment team, the second is consulting the guidelines, and the third is obtaining a formal second opinion from another doctor, either virtually or in person.

Here is a summary of the main items you should cover when deciding upon your treatment plan:

- ☐ I have discussed with my doctors the option of having an MDT review of my case.

- ☐ I have discussed with my doctors the option of having reviews of my pathology and radiology reports, if not done as part of an MDT discussion.

- ☐ I have read and understand the patient guidelines pertaining to my situation.

- ☐ I have read and understand the physician guidelines pertaining to my situation.

- ☐ I have considered the option of getting a second opinion, either in person or virtually.

Time to Focus on Treatment

We are now going to shift our focus. The next section of the book is geared toward getting top-notch treatment. In the next three chapters, I'll walk you through the three major treatment options for cancer—surgery, radiation, and systemic therapy—before focusing on clinical trials, getting good care after treatment is done, the specific approaches that might be helpful if there is no curative option, and finally, some of the myths and truths of cancer care.

Some of the upcoming chapters might not apply to your situation. For some patients, only one type of treatment (perhaps surgery) is required. If that's the case for you, then just focus on the relevant section. Start with the chapters that are most important to you now. For example, many women with breast cancer receive surgery, then systemic therapy, then radiation, in that order, and it would be most helpful to read the chapters in that same sequence.

Let's get started.

Resources

Accessing Treatment Guidelines

Standard Online Resources for Patients

Usually, the best place to start is with the National Comprehensive Cancer Network's Guidelines for Patients (http://www.nccn .org). The NCCN provides patient guideline booklets for more than 15 different types of cancers. These booklets discuss the diagnosis, the required tests for staging, and the treatment options. They are well written and easy to follow.

If the NCCN has a patient guideline book covering your type of cancer, read through it, and then move on to the advanced resources provided in the next section. If your type of cancer isn't covered in the NCCN booklets, the next place to look is Cancer.Net, a website run by the American Society of Clinical Oncology (ASCO). ASCO is an association of more than 40,000 oncology professionals from around the world and is widely considered to be the leading oncology organization in the world. Cancer.Net contains specific information on more than 150 different types of cancers.

Once you've read the patient-specific information, you can move on to the resources for doctors.

Online Resources for Doctors

As a patient, you can access the websites that doctors use to get detailed information about cancer treatment. Many doctors, including me, rely on these websites for our day-to-day practice. If I go to one of these websites and it tells me that the standard treatment option for a certain situation is to recommend chemotherapy and radiation, and if the site provides good evidence to back it up, then that becomes the default approach that I would consider. As we discussed in chapter 5, sometimes there are good reasons why treatment recommendations differ from guidelines, but the recommendations are a good place to start.

Don't be put off by the fact that these websites use medical terms. Even though you'll encounter medical jargon, you should be able to work your way through these sites. Use online medical dictionaries and the Patient Toolkit videos to guide you. Your doctor can also help walk you through them. Make sure you read the basic patient information websites that I listed above first so that you have a good background before starting. But don't be intimidated.

To carry on with our discussion of online resources for doctors, I'll present three resources: the overall NCCN Guidelines®, intended for physicians; the physician website UpToDate®; and the PubMed database.

NCCN Guidelines for Physicians

The NCCN has created physician guidelines for more than 40 types of cancer (https://www.nccn.org). These guidelines provide much more detailed information than the patient versions, and they are available free of charge (you just need to create an account on the NCCN website).

When you use the NCCN physician guides, the flowcharts take you step-by-step through the treatment approaches followed for each type of cancer, broken down by stage. There are also guidelines that cover cancer prevention, hereditary cancers, and supportive care for symptoms like nausea, pain, and fatigue.

UpToDate

Another excellent source of information is UpToDate (http://www.uptodate.com/home). This website provides physician-written articles on more than 10,000 topics, including hundreds of cancer-related topics. Each UpToDate article is an in-depth summary of a specific topic, written by physician experts in that field and updated frequently with the latest medical information.

Many physicians rely on UpToDate daily to help with their medical practice. If someone asks me a medical question and I don't know the answer, it's the first place I look. In my experience, it's the best medical knowledge tool available.

The downside to UpToDate is that it's not free. Physicians (including me) who want to use it pay for an annual subscription. Patients can access some specific patient information for free, but that material is limited to the basics. Fortunately, UpToDate offers short-term subscriptions, so you can get the information you need without having to pay for an annual subscription.

If you're not sure whether UpToDate will be worth the cost, you can search the database for free and buy only a short subscription once you find something that you'd like to read.

PubMed

This third resource is a very technical one and would be useful only if you really can't find information elsewhere. PubMed (https://www.pubmed.com) is a searchable database of research articles. It can be helpful if you have a *very* specific question that you can't find answers to elsewhere (and if your doctors can't answer it easily), but it's much too detailed for general information. For example, if you search for "breast cancer treatment," you get more than 170,000 articles. So don't use PubMed for the basics.

But if you have a specific question, it might be useful. If you search for articles with the words "fertility preservation options for breast cancer," you get a list of about 90 titles. You can then scan those titles quickly to see if any of them match what you are looking for. There are other tricks for making your searches more specific, and these are discussed in the video titled "Accessing Online Resources for Doctors" in the Patient Toolkit. Because PubMed is a highly technical resource, it is important to review any searches with your health care team, including your doctor. A cancer librarian can also be extremely helpful if you want to search PubMed.

When you find an article on PubMed, you can usually see the title and its *abstract,* a brief summary of its content, for free. In some cases, you can also read the whole article free of charge. But some of the journal articles require a paid subscription. There are often ways around having to pay; you can ask your cancer librarian to get an article for you, for example, or you can e-mail the author of the article asking for a free copy, or you can ask your doctor to get you a copy, as many doctors will have access through their institution.

Finding a Doctor

There are no blanket statements that can guarantee you will find a good doctor or hospital, but there are some helpful approaches you can take. Start by reading through the chapters of this book pertaining to the treatments that are relevant for your type of cancer. For example, if your type of cancer is often treated by surgery, read through chapter 9 to get an idea of some of the important factors in choosing a surgeon.

The American Cancer Society provides excellent, in-depth resources discussing many of the issues to consider in finding a doctor, including two useful worksheets: "How to Choose a Hospital" and "How to Choose a Doctor" (linked at http://www.quality cancertreatment.com/a06).

Some institutions in the United States and other countries provide rankings of hospitals based on wide-ranging criteria. Although the rankings can be controversial, they do provide helpful information, particularly if a hospital near you is ranked highly on different lists. The Leapfrog Group provides some very useful tools to get started, including a directory of hospital rankings and a "Hospital Safety Score" tool (both linked at http://www.qualitycan certreatment.com/a06).

Finally, in the United States, it is worth considering visiting a National Cancer Institute (NCI)–designated cancer center or a Commission on Cancer (CoC)–accredited program. The NCI designation applies to 69 centers across America (at the time of writing) that meet certain criteria (more details are available at http://cancercenters.cancer.gov/Center/CancerCenters). And the CoC, of the American College of Surgeons, accredits cancer programs that meet prespecified standards (see http://www.facs.org/search /cancer-programs).

In addition to the expertise of your doctor, it's important to consider your doctor's interactions with you:

- Does he seem organized?

- Did he take a proper medical history at first consultation?

- Is he attentive when you are asking questions?

- Does he answer your questions effectively? Has he anticipated all your questions in a way that gives you confidence that he's had this discussion many times and fully understands your disease?

- Does he have a good understanding of your test results?

- Did he properly inform you of the treatment options, risks, and benefits?

- Does he ask about your individual values and preferences?

- Does he follow up on tests and appointments, or does he forget to arrange them, leaving you to call the office and remind his staff?

Your doctor needs to understand your medical situation in detail, assess your risks (which are based on your medical history and your answers to questions), give you a balanced view of the risks and benefits, and coordinate important tests and appointments, both before and after treatment. You need to be confident that things will not be missed.

Getting
World-Class
Care

CHAPTER 9

Getting Top-Notch Surgery

You've decided that surgery is the right treatment for you. You call your surgeon to tell her that you're ready to go.

Not so fast, I would say. You shouldn't just decide, *I want to have surgery.* Rather, you should decide, *I want to have the best surgery possible and maximize my chance of cure.*

Surgery is a major weapon in the fight against cancer, and it has helped to cure millions of patients with cancer around the world. But surgery is inherently risky and complex, and for these reasons, your decision to have surgery is different from almost any other big decision in your life.

By comparison, let's imagine that you've decided to buy a new car. You would research different models of cars, looking at things like reliability, safety, performance, and cost. You would test-drive a few models and then decide on a new car that is right for you. You could buy that model at any dealership in your area or across the country, and your car would be essentially the same. Most other purchases in life are like this: they are mass-produced, and the quality is standardized. But when the "product" is surgery, the quality is more variable because it is performed by a team of individuals.

The quality of your surgery—and your chance of success—depends on who does your surgery, where it is done, and the safety procedures in place at that hospital. The impact is big. In some cases, your chance of survival can be more than doubled. The more complicated the surgery, the more the results can vary.

This raises some important questions: How big are these differences, and why do they arise? By understanding these issues, you can make sure that you get the best possible surgery.

When you want to book a vacation, you can go to a website with thousands of hotel reviews to help you make your choice. When you are buying a car, you can take it one step further: after reading reviews, you can actually go to a car lot and experience the car for yourself by taking a test-drive. Reviews of a surgeon's operating skills are not available, and there's no option for a test-drive. So how can you be sure that you are getting good surgical care? You need to take a close look at your hospital and your surgeon.

The Importance of Hospital Volume

When patients with head and neck cancer come for their first visit at the cancer center where I work, they get a two-for-one deal: they meet me (or another radiation oncologist) and a head and neck cancer surgeon at the same time, in the same examination room. With both of us there, we discuss the options for treatment. This setup provides them with two opinions at once, and it is part of providing good-quality care.[*]

If surgery is in the cards, the surgeon will carefully explain the surgery and the risks and benefits. Occasionally, a patient will ask, sometimes with a nervous laugh, "Have you done this surgery before?" The patient is looking for reassurance that his operation will not be the surgeon's first attempt at that procedure. It seems like a reasonable question. Patients want to know the level of experience of their surgeon, and this is an important issue that we will discuss more later.

---

[*] These types of clinics are called "multidisciplinary clinics," and many centers run them for various types of cancer. They allow patients to obtain opinions from multiple specialists at once, helping to ensure that patients are aware of all options.

But the question that no one ever asks is: "How many times a year does your hospital do this procedure?" The answer to this—the *hospital volume*—can have a big impact on your chances of surviving the surgery. I've never heard a patient ask that question.

Surgeon John Birkmeyer is a pioneer in the study of the factors that affect surgical outcomes, and he has revolutionized our understanding of the best ways to deliver cancer care. In a landmark article published in the prestigious *New England Journal of Medicine*, Dr. Birkmeyer and his team looked at the relationship between the hospital volume—the number of procedures done in a hospital per year—and the risk of dying after surgery.[60]

Birkmeyer's team looked at 14 types of surgeries, including 8 cancer surgeries, in about 2.5 million US Medicare patients. The results for the highest-volume hospitals—those doing these surgeries the most frequently—are shown in table 3.

Table 3. Patient Survival in Highest-Volume Hospitals

Type of Cancer Surgery	Hospital Volume (surgeries per year)	Risk of Dying from Surgery
Bladder	>11	3%
Colon	>124	4%
Esophagus	>19	8%
Kidney	>31	2%
Lobe of lung	>46	4%
Pancreas	>16	4%
Stomach	>21	9%
Whole lung	>46	11%

This table tells us that in hospitals where more than 124 patients per year have a *colectomy*—the removal of the colon—for cancer treatment, the risk of dying either within 30 days of surgery or before discharge home is 4 in 100. Removal of the whole lung (*pneumonectomy*) carries a higher risk. In hospitals that carry out more than 46 of these lung surgeries per year, the risk of death is 11 in 100.

What do we learn from this data from the highest-volume hospitals? Three important things.

First, cancer surgery comes with a risk, and that risk depends on the type of surgery. Removal of the kidney (2 percent risk of death) is less risky than removing the stomach (9 percent) or whole lung (11 percent).

Second, at high-volume centers, death after surgery is not very common for most procedures, usually with a risk that is less than 5 percent (which is equal to 1 in 20). While any risk of death should be minimized, some risk is unavoidable. But this risk should always be weighed against the benefits of surgery, as we discussed in chapter 7. If the benefit of undergoing the surgery is a good chance of prolonging your life, improving your symptoms, or curing your cancer, then the surgery is usually worthwhile. But if those benefits don't outweigh the risks, then surgery should be reconsidered.

Third, we learn from this table that some hospitals do very high volumes of surgery. Hospitals doing 125 colectomies or more per year are doing more than two per week on average. With those numbers, the doctors, nurses, and other team members are quite accustomed to dealing with these surgeries and managing the potential complications.

Now let's look at the results at the lowest-volume hospitals, where these surgeries are uncommon.

Table 4. Patient Survival in Low-Volume Hospitals

Type of Cancer Surgery	Hospital Volume (surgeries per year)	Risk of Dying	Additional Deaths per 100 Patients (compared with high-volume hospitals)
Bladder	<2	6%	3
Colon	<33	6%	2
Esophagus	<2	20%	12
Kidney	<7	3%	1
Lobe of lung	<9	6%	2
Pancreas	<1	16%	12
Stomach	<5	11%	2
Whole lung	<9	16%	5

Compare the results in table 4 with those in table 3. Some of the differences are sobering. In hospitals where, on average, fewer than 2 patients per year have their esophagus removed for cancer, 20 percent of patients will die—that's 1 in 5! By comparison, in the first table, that risk of death was only 8 percent. That means that for every 100 patients who have surgery at the lowest-volume hospitals, 12 more will die after surgery. The differences are also dramatic for other procedures: 12 more would die per 100 surgeries for removal of the pancreas (*pancreatectomy*); 5 more would die per 100 surgeries for removal of the whole lung; and there are smaller but still important differences for the rest.

Hundreds of studies have now examined the relationship between hospital volumes and mortality. It is clear that for many types of surgeries (although not all), higher volumes lead to better outcomes.[61]

Why do these differences exist? There is no single factor, but it is essentially the notion that "practice makes perfect." High-volume hospitals have more experienced staff. They have dealt with surgical complications numerous times before and are probably more adept at recognizing problems early, before they become life-threatening. High-volume hospitals often have better infrastructure and resources. It can be very helpful to have a variety of specialists and an intensive care unit available when there is a complication. For example, if a patient has a heart attack after surgery, it can be critically important to have a cardiologist on-site to see the patient immediately. If she has a severe infection, a specialist in infectious diseases can be called.

Given the importance of hospital volume, it's often important to find out whether your surgery will occur at a low-volume or high-volume center. Depending on where you live, you might be able to find information about local hospital volumes online, and some websites are listed in the resources at the end of this chapter. Unfortunately, many hospitals will not have this information easily available online. You should then ask your surgeon: "How many of these surgeries are performed at this hospital every year?" If the number sounds low, ask your surgeon to discuss the importance of hospital volume for the type of surgery that you are having and whether other hospitals—nearby or elsewhere—have higher volumes.*

---

* You can use the tables above to show you what "high-volume" means for those types of surgeries.

Your Choice of Surgeon

Hospitals are not created equal, and neither are surgeons. Surgery is an extremely complicated task, and some surgeons perform better than others. A surgeon doing a difficult operation needs to integrate anatomy knowledge, dexterity, visual and tactile cues, and judgment, all in real time. The surgeon needs to be a strong communicator and leader in the operating room. Not only are these tasks difficult, but they must sometimes be done in a stressful situation. Although most of the time, the operating room is relatively calm, a crisis can arise quickly, and those emergencies often require a decisive response and grace under pressure.

Surgeons differ in their level of training and experience. If you need to have part of your colon removed, a general surgeon could do it for you. He would have completed a residency that trains him to do a wide variety of surgeries, including colon removal. Alternatively, you could have it done by a colorectal surgeon, who has completed extra training after a general surgery residency to further focus on surgery of the colon and rectum. Similarly, if you are having your lung or esophagus removed, it could be done by a general surgeon, or it could be done by a thoracic surgeon, who has undergone even more specialty training to learn more about operating inside the chest.

In both situations, the more specialization the better. For colorectal cancer surgery, patients operated on by general surgeons have a much higher risk—three times higher—of the cancer coming back in the same area compared with patients operated on by colorectal surgeons.[62] For lung cancer surgery, the risk of dying from surgery is 1–2 percent lower if a thoracic surgeon is doing the operation compared with a general surgeon.[63]

In addition to training, the number of surgeries performed per year by your surgeon is also a very important factor. Similar to the findings with hospital volumes, surgeons who perform operations more frequently confer better survival rates, even at high-volume hospitals. For some cancers, the differences in the risk of dying are relatively small (1 more patient dying per 100 for lung cancer surgeries, comparing the lowest-volume and highest-volume surgeons), but for others, they are large (10 more patients dying per 100 for pancreatic or esophageal cancer).[64]

Depending on the type of surgery, it may take hundreds of surgeries for a cancer surgeon to be at her best. A study of almost 8,000 men who underwent removal of the prostate (*prostatectomy*) found that the best results were obtained by surgeons after they completed at least 250 surgeries. The chances of the cancer returning were lowest (10.7 percent) above that threshold of 250 surgeries and highest (17.9 percent) when the surgeon had done only 10.[65]

The more complicated the task, the longer it can take to become proficient. *Minimally invasive surgery* (MIS) is one example. MIS is a type of surgery in which instead of making a large incision, small incisions are used and the surgeons work with special cameras and tools. For a man having a minimally invasive prostatectomy, surgeons may require as many as 750 surgeries to be at their best.[66] A similar problem may be seen with the use of robotic surgery, where the surgeon is using special cameras and tools but also operating them using robotic controls.

Not all surgeries take so long to learn to do extremely well, but it's clear that surgical experience is very important. Sometimes new technologies provide important benefits, but sometimes they do not. Being one of the first patients to undergo a new, complicated procedure, such as MIS or robotic surgery, might come with additional risks because your surgeon is still learning.

So which is more important: the hospital you choose or the surgeon you choose? Most studies that have looked at both factors suggest that the surgical volumes have the biggest impact.[67] So the priority for most patients should be to find a high-volume surgeon. But the best scenario is to find a high-volume surgeon at a high-volume hospital.

There is one clear downside to this approach. If everyone chose only an experienced, high-volume surgeon to do their surgery, how would we train any new doctors? We need a continual supply of new surgeons to replace those who are retiring or who are too busy to increase their workloads. Every surgeon must start with his or her first case. One solution to this problem is to ensure that the newbies have appropriate training and backup supports. This starts with specialty training, whereby young surgeons undertake increasingly complex surgeries at a center of excellence, under the supervision of an experienced mentor. When training is finished and the surgeon starts working independently, more experienced colleagues can be an asset: if the new surgeon runs into an unforeseen issue, he can call a colleague to join him in the operating room.

You should also be aware of a related issue: experienced, high-volume surgeons will often have young trainees assisting at surgery. Top surgeons at well-known centers are sought out by trainees looking to improve their surgical knowledge and beef up their résumés. Trainees are crucial, and many studies suggest that being treated at *academic hospitals* (hospitals that include teaching) is good. But you don't want a situation in which you go to a top-notch surgeon only to have your surgery done by an unsupervised trainee. Ask your surgeon: "If trainees are involved, will you be in the room supervising for the duration of the operation?" No meaningful operation can occur without assistants, and all surgeons need someone to help them, but you do want the main surgeon present and engaged in the entire process.

Surgical Checklists

Carrying out a successful surgery involves multiple important steps. The right patient has to be brought to the operating room, prepared properly for the surgery, and given the right medications. That person's medical case must be reviewed, and the team discusses their surgical approach. After the surgery, instruments have to be counted and medications or fluids have to be given. Skipping one of these steps can increase the risk of a complication and, in some cases, can lead to serious harm. Human memory is not perfect, and sometimes steps are missed.

In day-to-day life, we use checklists and to-do lists to keep ourselves organized, for simple things like grocery shopping and for complicated things like moving into a new house. For pilots, for whom a small mistake can have disastrous consequences, checklists are an important safety tool. Prior to takeoff, pilots and copilots work through a list of items, checking instruments, lights, and fuel. There are actually several checklists used during each flight and separate checklists to be used in cases of in-flight emergencies. When pilots forget to use the checklist or skip an item, accidents can occur. Kenneth Funk, PhD, an associate professor at Oregon State University, estimates that about 1 in 10 aviation accidents are related to a missed item on a checklist, using the wrong checklist, or using a checklist improperly.[68]

Can surgeons learn from pilots? Absolutely. In 2008, the World Health Organization and researchers from Harvard University developed and evaluated a 19-point checklist to be used before surgery to reduce the risk of major complications.[69] The checklist includes items to be done before the patient is put to sleep (such as confirming the patient identity, marking the site of surgery, checking the anesthesia machine), before the incision (identifying all team members by name, making sure antibiotics have been given, confirming instruments are sterile), and before the patient leaves the operating room (counting tools and sponges, identifying concerns for patient recovery).*

The checklist was tested at eight hospitals around the world, including locations in Canada, India, Jordan, New Zealand, the Philippines, Tanzania, England, and the United States.[70] The authors compared results from approximately 3,700 surgeries done before the checklist was implemented and 4,000 surgeries done after. The results were impressive. After implementation of the checklist, there were significant improvements in several surgical outcomes, including the risk of surgical death, complication rates, postoperative infection rates, and the risk of the patient needing an unplanned reoperation to address a complication.

Why does the checklist work? The obvious answer is that it makes sure no steps are missed. More importantly, though, it changes the hospital procedures for the better. Giving antibiotics just prior to surgery is key to reducing the risk of postoperative infection. Instead of giving preoperative antibiotics on the ward—where staff are busy and doses can be missed—the antibiotics are given in the operating room, and the checklist ensures they are not missed. The checklist also changes the attitudes and behaviors of the surgical team. As part of the list, all staff members identify themselves by name, reinforcing their ability to speak up in case there are problems. Before and after the surgery, the checklist includes a debriefing, wherein patient-specific concerns are discussed aloud.

Several other studies support the notion that surgical checklists improve outcomes.[71] But not all studies show this effect.[72] The value of the checklists probably depends on several factors, including how

---

* You can download the checklist at http://www.who.int/patientsafety/safesurgery/ ss_checklist/en/.

well the team functions before the checklists are introduced (well-functioning teams may not improve much more) and whether team-building and proper training exercises are completed as well.

The benefits of checklists are not confined to the operating room. Just as pilots use separate checklists for different phases of the flight and for emergencies, doctors do the same for different phases of the hospital stay. Researchers have expanded the surgical checklist to include the time in hospital before and after surgery, and they have created separate checklists for emergencies that occur in the operating room, such as major bleeding or cardiac arrest. These checklists have also improved patient outcomes and physician performance.[73]

The data supporting checklists is compelling and has had an impact. In a survey of operating room staff who had implemented the surgical safety checklist, 93 percent indicated they would want the checklist used if they were having an operation.[74] In the study testing checklists for crisis situations that can occur during surgery, 97 percent of participants reported that they would want the checklist used if such an emergency happened during one of their operations.[75]

If doctors and operating staff would want checklists used during their surgery, so should you. Ask your surgeon if her team uses safety checklists and whether they use checklists before or after surgery as well.

Out of Surgery, Not Out of the Woods

Most of the time, surgical complications don't arise during the surgery itself but afterward. Your care in the hospital after surgery plays an important role in your chances of success. Often new medical issues arise, like infections or low blood counts, and need to be addressed by the team. You will often be placed on new medications. Blood work might be done daily, and you might undergo additional imaging, such as chest X-rays or CT scans. There are several other things that you can help keep track of during your hospital admission.

The Team

Get to know the names of the members of your surgical team, including any residents or trainees. They may be the ones doing rounds on you every day. Make sure they know who your family contact is. Find out what time the team will be making rounds and make sure your contact can be present to hear the plan for the day, get the update on your progress, and ask any questions you might have.

Test Results

Just as you've learned to collect and interpret your medical records in chapter 4, you can do the same while in the hospital. You can ask for copies of all imaging tests and oral or written results from abnormal blood work. Ask your team if you have questions about a result.

Medications

If new any medications are added to your medication list or medications are discontinued, ask your team to explain the underlying reasons. Obtaining your full medication list will give you a good idea of the current issues and how they are being treated. Also, if you are having symptoms like pain or nausea, you will know which medications are already ordered to be taken as needed.

Vital Signs

Your nurse will be checking your vital signs on a regular basis. Your vital signs include your heart rate, breathing rate, temperature, and blood pressure. If some of your vitals are off (like your blood pressure being low or your temperature being high), ask why and ask how the team is looking after that issue.

Preventive Steps

There are also some key preventive steps your team should take that can reduce the risk of serious complications, and you can help by double-checking that they are done. Often patients are given antibiotics immediately before surgery to prevent the risk of infection, and blood thinners after surgery to reduce the risk of blood clots. Catheters are removed when no longer needed, to prevent infection. In many situations, getting up and walking shortly after surgery helps recovery. You can print out one of the safety checklists, bring it with you to the hospital, and ask your team to go through it with you.* Of course, during your stay, report any new symptoms to your team immediately, like new pain or fever.

Handwashing

Poor hand hygiene by hospital staff is a contributing factor to the spread of hospital infections.[76] Sadly, doctors can be the least compliant staff members when it comes to handwashing recommendations.[77] Ask your nurse to put a bottle of hand sanitizer gel at your bedside, or put one there yourself. Whenever a team member comes to see you (whether it's a doctor, nurse, or any other staff), politely ask if they've had a chance to clean their hands.

---

* The name of the checklist that covers a complete surgical admission to the hospital is SURPASS, and you can download it at http://www.surpass-checklist.nl. Since it's posted on a Dutch website, you first have to choose English as your language, then use the "Download SURPASS checklist" link.

Wrap-up and Mini-checklist

In this chapter, you've learned that outcomes from surgery vary immensely, depending on the hospital and surgeon. Practice makes perfect, and surgeons who are better trained, who work at high-volume hospitals, who have high-volume practices, and who use checklists tend to have better outcomes.

Is this all worth the effort? Should you switch hospitals or surgeons based on the factors we've discussed here? It is a decision worth considering and discussing with your doctors. You have to weigh many factors in your decision, including travel logistics, distance from home, and whether your insurance or government will pay for treatment at the other hospital. But the benefit appears to be large for many surgeries and should not be ignored.

To put these numbers in perspective, let's look at the amount of benefit provided by chemotherapy for lung cancer. Many lung cancer patients will go through four months of chemotherapy after surgery because it improves their chances of cure. For every 100 patients who get that chemotherapy, 5 extra patients will be alive after five years because of the chemotherapy.[18] Those four months of chemotherapy can be difficult, but to most people, it is worthwhile for a 5 percent improvement in survival. Switching to a high-volume hospital or surgeon might provide an equal or larger benefit for much less effort.

Here is a checklist of the key questions for your surgeon covering the important issues, including some of the relevant questions discussed in earlier chapters:

☐ *Even though you are recommending surgery, are there any other alternative treatments available?*

If the answer is yes, then you should ask:

• *How do you know that surgery is better than these other options?*

- *Can I meet with those specialists (such as a radiation doctor) to discuss those alternatives?*

☐ *Will I need other treatments after surgery (like chemotherapy and radiation)?*

If the answer is yes, then ask:

- *What is the added benefit of surgery over just having these other treatments?*

☐ *What is your training background? Are you board-certified, and do you have specialty training?*

☐ *Are you considered a high-volume surgeon for this type of procedure, and is this considered a high-volume hospital? How many of these surgeries are done by you and your team each year?**

☐ *Do you use surgical safety checklists?*

☐ *Do you have data reporting your own surgical outcomes, including rates of complications and survival?*

☐ *What kind of backup is available if there is an unexpected issue, either during my surgery or afterward? For example, if I have a serious lung or heart issue, are there appropriate specialists and an intensive care unit on-site, or would I need to be transferred elsewhere?*

- *If trainees are involved, will you be in the room and supervising for the duration of my surgery?*

---

* A USA *Today* article provides a good list of questions to ask regarding low-volume hospitals (linked at http://www.qualitycancertreatment.com/a07).

Resources

Hospital Volume

The easiest way to find out about hospital volumes and surgeon volumes is just to ask your individual surgeon. Online information can be sparse, but there are a few helpful websites available, particularly in the United States. Many of them are available through the Leapfrog Group (either provided by Leapfrog or listed in its directory of resources; see http://www.qualitycancertreatment.com/a06 for the links). These include Medicare's Hospital Compare website and the Hospital Safety Grade website (both of which are also linked at http://www.qualitycancertreatment.com/a06). These sites compare hospitals in several categories, including whether important steps are taken to make surgery safer and reduce complication rates.

CHAPTER 10

Is Your Radiation Hit-or-Miss?

For patients, radiation treatment is the most mysterious part of cancer care. It can be difficult to understand exactly what is happening, and it's not obvious whether you're getting good treatment or not.

First, the staff call your name and you are led down a twisting hallway into a special shielded room with a big radiation machine. You lie down on a hard table. Special devices are used to prevent you from wiggling—sometimes it's a mask that goes over your face and attaches to the table, and sometimes it's a special vacuum bag that is molded to the shape of your body. Once you are in position, the overhead lights dim and you see colored laser beams throughout the room. The therapists move you and the table into position, lining up the lasers with some dots they've marked on your body. They leave. You wait.

The radiation machine moves around you and makes some noises. It pauses, then makes some more noises. You usually don't feel a thing.

Eventually, the machine stops, the lights come on, and you walk out. You're done for the day. The process repeats itself, often daily (usually only on weekdays) for several weeks.

The mystery lies in the fact that as a patient, you have no way of knowing exactly where the radiation is going, how much radiation is hitting the tumor, and how much is hitting your healthy normal tissues. You trust your health care team to make sure that everything is done correctly. For most patients, there is no double-checking.

Radiation is a valuable weapon in the fight against cancer. Radiation, on its own, can cure many types of cancer, including cancers of the prostate, lung, skin, head and neck, and cervix.[79] Sometimes radiation is combined with chemotherapy to enhance its tumor-killing effect and improve the chances of cure. Other times, radiation plays a supporting role when surgery is the main treatment—it can be given before surgery, to shrink down a tumor, or after surgery, to mop up any leftover cancer cells. Many women with breast cancer can avoid a mastectomy by having breast-conserving surgery (a *lumpectomy*) followed by radiation. The radiation makes up for the fact that the smaller surgery might leave some cancer cells behind.

Properly designed and delivered, radiation is a powerful tool that has saved countless lives. In a carefully designed treatment with good quality control, the tumor gets a high dose of radiation while the amount of radiation delivered to healthy tissues is minimized.

But radiation can be a double-edged sword. Too much radiation to healthy tissues, or too little radiation to the tumor, can have disastrous consequences.[80] A small error, resulting in a radiation dose that is off by 1 percent from what is prescribed or in positioning that is off by a few millimeters, is likely to be inconsequential. But a major error, such as failing to treat an area of tumor, could leave a patient with no chance of cure.

With radiation treatment, there are rarely any second chances. If the tumor doesn't receive enough radiation the first time around, it can be very hard to go back later and add more safely. If the normal healthy tissues receive too much radiation, there is no eraser to remove the radiation that's been given.

This chapter is meant to shed some light on the process of radiation treatment for cancer. You will learn how to double-check that you are receiving the correct dose of radiation and that your radiation treatment is designed safely. In order to do this, you first need to understand some of the background information: What is radiation, and how are treatments designed?

An Invisible Cancer-Killing Beam

Radiation is an invisible beam that can kill cancer cells. You can't see it, smell it, or feel it while it's being delivered (but you can feel the effects of it afterward, as side effects can develop over the course of treatment). You can think of radiation as an invisible beam of light, like a flashlight, that can penetrate the body and hit the cancer cells.

Usually, the radiation used to treat cancer is a beam of X-rays, just like the X-rays that are used to take a chest X-ray, but more powerful. When you turn on a flashlight, the beam of light that comes out is made of up *photons*—millions of little packets of light. When we use X-rays to treat cancer, we also call them photons. The vast majority of patients who receive radiation are treated with photons, but there are also other types of radiation available that are made up of very small particles, including *electrons, protons,* and more rarely, *neutrons.* We'll discuss these different types of radiation later in the chapter. For most patients, the type of radiation (whether it's photons, electrons, or protons) is not nearly as relevant as the amount of radiation that they receive, or the *dose.*

When doctors prescribe medicine to their patients, the drug dose is usually measured in *milligrams* (mg), which is a small unit of mass, telling how much the drug weighs. If you have an infection, your doctor might prescribe 500 mg of penicillin. If you are getting chemotherapy, you might get 150 mg of the drug cisplatin.

We can't prescribe radiation in milligrams because it has no mass that we can measure. The units that we use to measure radiation are called *Gray* (Gy), which tells us how much radiation is absorbed by the body. To give you some context for these units, consider the fact that we all get exposed to some radiation as part of normal day-to-day living (from sources like the sun, food, air, and minerals in the earth). This *background radiation* amounts to the equivalent of only about 0.002 Gy per year in most places. When you get a chest X-ray, you receive a small dose, about 0.0001 Gy.[81] When we treat cancer, the doses of radiation needed to cure a cancer are much higher, often in the range of 60–70 Gy, depending on the type of cancer.

Radiation is usually not given all at once. We tend to give radiation little by little, day by day, in *fractions*, or smaller doses. Many patients receive one fraction of 2 Gy each day, five days per week. This works out to 10 Gy per week. For a six-week treatment, that would be 60 Gy and a total of 30 fractions.

We give the radiation in small daily fractions for a few reasons. First, if we gave all the radiation at once, it would be very toxic, even lethal. Second, these small doses take advantage of some of the differences between normal cells and tumor cells, such as the fact that normal cells are better able to repair the damage from the radiation overnight between treatments, whereas tumor cells can't repair the damage as well.

The number of fractions prescribed is also important for a few reasons. The number can determine if a treatment has the potential to cure the cancer or not. For most cancers, a dose of 30 Gy in 10 fractions (3 Gy per day over two weeks) cannot cure a cancer, but it could shrink it and improve some symptoms. This type of dose is used in a palliative setting. But 30 Gy given in a single fraction—all at once—is an extremely potent dose of radiation that can be used (with the proper equipment) in an attempt to cure certain cancers. The number of fractions makes a big difference for potency.

The other reason that the number of fractions is important is a practical one: sometimes doctors can give radiation over a shorter period of time with the same effect, if they give a slightly larger daily dose. When this is possible, treatment times can be shortened by a few weeks, which is much more convenient for patients.

Here are some examples of how shorter treatment spans can be convenient yet just as effective as longer treatments. For women with breast cancer who have had a lumpectomy and need radiation, a five-week course of radiation (2 Gy per day for 25 fractions, for a total of 50 Gy) was the standard for many years. But a shorter treatment, only three weeks plus one day, works just as well (2.66 Gy per day for 16 fractions, for a total of 42.5 Gy) without more side effects.[82] This saves each woman nine trips to the cancer center. Note that the total dose was reduced from 50 Gy to 42.5 Gy when the treatment was shortened, to keep the risk of side effects the same. For many patients who have painful spots of cancer in their bones, a single dose of 8 Gy works just as well as a two-week (or longer) treatment, again saving nine visits.[83] The single treatment is especially convenient for patients: in some cases, they can see the doctor and get their radiation all in the same day.

The first thing you need to double-check about your radiation is the dose and the number of fractions. Ask your doctor:

- *What is the dose and fractionation of radiation that you are prescribing, and is it standard for this situation?*

  Standard radiation doses for most types of cancer are listed in the resources at the end of chapter 8 (such as the NCCN physician guidelines).

- *Can my treatment be delivered in a smaller number of fractions and still have the same benefits and the same risks of side effects?*

The Design Process

Before you start your radiation, a radiation plan has to be designed for you. In most cases, your doctor will arrange for a CT *simulation,* which is a special type of CT scan specifically used for radiation planning. You will often receive tattoos (small dots on your skin) that are used to help position you. Your doctor might also use an immobilization device, such as a custom mask for head and neck radiation, to keep you positioned correctly.

After the scan is complete, there are dozens of tasks that need to be done correctly behind the scenes to make sure that everything turns out as intended. The doctor in charge of your radiation, the radiation oncologist, looks at the CT simulation scan and outlines the areas of known cancer, along with any areas at risk of having cancer (such as lymph nodes). To do this, the doctor uses drawing tools on a computer program (such as a pencil tool) to trace around the borders of the tumor. In the same way, using the drawing tools, the doctor (or other team members) will outline the healthy normal tissues that need to be avoided.

After the outlining is done, a *dosimetrist*—a radiation planner—designs a radiation plan based on those outlines. Properly designed radiation plans are like nice paintings, with all the brushstrokes in the right places, and these top-quality radiation plans can be very elegant, as you'll see below. But improperly designed plans are a problem. They can lead to lower chances of cure[84] or higher chances of side effects.[85] Some of these issues have been highlighted in media reports, including a 2010 series in the *New York Times.** The radiation machine knows where to put the radiation—and where not to put it—only because of human input. If an area of tumor is not outlined, the radiation plan won't aim to treat it. And if a normal organ isn't outlined, the plan won't try to avoid it.

---

*   This newspaper series is linked at http://www.qualitycancertreatment.com/a01.

Figure 6 shows an example of a radiation treatment plan, to illustrate how complicated it can be (you can view a color version of this figure at http://qualitycancertreatment.com/links). There is another sample radiation plan, with a video explanation, available in the online Patient Toolkit (at http://www.qualitycancertreatment.com /toolkit).

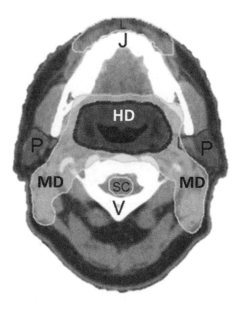

Figure 6. Radiation Treatment Plan for a Head and Neck Cancer

You can easily see the jaw (J) and one of the bones of the spine (a *vertebra*, V). The high dose area (HD) treats where the cancer is known to be, and the medium dose area (MD) treats areas where the cancer might be. But you can also see the areas that are being avoided by the bulk of the radiation, including the lips (L), the salivary glands (the *parotids*, P), and the spinal cord (SC). These are only a few of the important areas. For head and neck cancer radiation plans, there are more than 20 different structures to try to avoid, including the eyes, the brain, important nerves, hearing organs, and swallowing muscles.

Safety Should Be the First Priority

Even though radiation is complex, with the proper checks and audits in place, it can be made to be very safe. These safety measures include double-checking the patient identification, the location and outlining of the tumor, the radiation design, patient positioning, and the performance of the treatment machines. Among top-notch centers, radiation safety is a major priority. Many of the national and international radiation oncology centers have task forces and provide recommendations about radiation safety. But even with the recommendations available, some radiation centers will be more committed than others, with more safety checks in place.

As a patient, you are not expected to double-check that every single step is being done correctly. But by asking the right questions, you can find out whether many of the important safety checks are in place at your institution. In the rest of this chapter, we will review the key issues to ask about.

Peer Review and Other Important Checks

Many radiation oncology teams—but certainly not all—conduct *quality assurance rounds* or *chart rounds:* special meetings to confirm treatment plans. At these meetings, radiation oncologists and dosimetrists provide second opinions specifically on radiation treatment plans. The group briefly discusses the patient's clinical situation, then reviews elements of the treatment plan, including the structures that have been outlined and the doses delivered to those structures. This type of peer review can have a big impact: approximately one out of every nine radiation plans that are reviewed undergo a change. More than half of the time, the changes relate to issues with the delineation of the target itself.[86]

I attend peer review rounds for two hours every week. I review the radiation treatment plans created by my colleagues and they review mine. When we first initiated this practice, I lamented the fact that so much of my time would be spent on peer review, taking away from time to see patients or do research. I didn't think that big problems would be found. But over time, I found that occasionally, big issues are found and corrected. I now believe that peer review is essential.

In addition to the peer review, further checks by other team members are important. These team members include a *medical physicist* (a staff member with advanced physics certification) and a *radiation therapist* (a staff member who delivers radiation, also called a *radiotherapist* or *radiographer*), who can help catch errors.[87]

Ask your doctor if your radiation plan is peer-reviewed and if it's also checked again by a medical physicist and a radiation therapist. Your radiation oncologist should be able to describe the types of quality assurance checks that are done in his or her facility by the radiation team.

Expertise Is Important

As we discussed with surgery in chapter 9, practice makes perfect. The more often a surgeon does an operation, the better the outcomes are. For patients undergoing radiation, emerging data indicates that the same relationship holds true. We now have data from a few different types of cancers showing that patients who receive their radiation at high-volume centers have better outcomes.[88] As one author concluded when referring to radiation: "Centers treating only a few patients are the major source of quality problems."[89]

Ask your radiation doctor: "Is this considered to be a high-volume center for my type of cancer, and are you personally considered a high-volume doctor?"

Machines and Technology Are Less Important

There is an arms race under way in the field of radiation oncology. Companies and cancer centers are racing to develop, implement, and advertise the newest technologies. Many of these new machines have great-sounding names: CyberKnife®, Gamma Knife®, and TrueBeam™ are just a few. These machines all sound a lot more exciting than being treated on a "linear accelerator" (a generic name for many radiation machines).

To complicate matters further, the type of radiation can also vary. Most of these machines use photons or electrons, which have been used to treat cancer for many decades. Other centers advertise that they have newer particles that they claim are even better—you might hear about protons or, more rarely, carbon ions or neutrons.

How can you sort through all of these competing messages? Which machine and type of radiation should you choose? An in-depth technical review of all of these different machines wouldn't be useful and might be out-of-date only a few months after being written. But here is a high-level overview, with tips on four key issues: radiation design, image guidance, the radiation machine, and the use of protons.

The Radiation Design

Modern radiation is often designed using the process *intensity-modulated radiation therapy* (IMRT). IMRT is better at shaping the radiation beams than older techniques. In essence, while older radiation beams can be considered like a flashlight that is turned on and off, IMRT beams can be considered more like a grid of 100 tiny flashlights that can be individually turned on and off depending on the shape of the target.

In some cases, IMRT has proven beneficial for reducing side effects in randomized trials (as for head and neck cancer),[90] but in other cases, it may be a waste of time and resources. It is worth asking if IMRT is being used in your case and, if not, whether it would be beneficial.

Image Guidance

Another important capability is *image guidance,* which is using imaging to make sure the tumor is properly targeted. For some people with cancers being treated close to critical areas (like the spinal cord) or people being treated for cancers where movement of the tumor is of concern (some lung cancers), having image guidance capabilities can be essential for high-quality treatment. For example, most radiation machines now have the ability to acquire a form of CT scan prior to treatment to accurately verify a person's position before treatment. In other cases, a simple X-ray-like image can be taken to verify position. Like IMRT, some types of image guidance might not be necessary for all cases, and it is worth asking what type of image guidance is being used for your treatment.

The Radiation Machine

Modern radiation machines go by many different names, and radiation centers often advertise the name of the brand of machine that they have purchased. However, all modern radiation machines can produce excellent radiation plans, using IMRT or other techniques when necessary. There is very little clinical data suggesting superiority of one type of modern radiation machine over another, provided that they have similar general capabilities for IMRT and image guidance. No one has proven that any of the brands are better than any others when it comes to patient outcomes.

Protons or Photons

Proton therapy is widely advertised in some countries, including within the United States. Protons have some theoretical advantages over the standard photons because they might reduce the dose of radiation to normal organs, and therefore, they might reduce the side effects. As a result, they are most commonly used for children's cancers, where the risk of long-term side effects is highest. But there are also some potential disadvantages. Whether protons are better than photons is a matter of intense debate. As of now, only one randomized trial has compared protons and photons (for lung cancer) and found no difference.[91] Research is ongoing.

The overall message is this: machines and technology are probably not a big player in overall outcomes of cancer treatment, as long as the treatment machines are relatively modern. Other factors appear to be much more important, such as overall patient volumes, expertise, and the quality assurance process. Here are some questions to ask:

- *Would I be treated with photons, protons, or something else? Why do you feel that approach would be best for me?*

- *Will I be treated with IMRT? If not, would it be useful in my case?*

- *How modern is your radiation treatment machine? Do you think it matters whether I'm treated on this machine or another one?*

- *Does the equipment you have allow you to give the dose of radiation I need in the safest fashion possible?*

Reviewing Your Own Radiation Plan

Reviewing your radiation plan with your doctor can be very useful. It will help you to understand your radiation treatment and the potential side effects, and it serves as a mechanism to help double-check that you are getting high-quality care.

In this section, we'll go over the basic elements of reviewing the radiation plan. In the Patient Toolkit online (http://www.qualitycan certreatment.com/toolkit), you can watch videos that walk you through some radiation plans for different types of cancer. Most of this section will be applicable to radiation plans that are designed to try to cure the cancer (curative-intent treatments), in which we prescribe the highest doses. When we use radiation for palliative treatments, we tend to use lower doses, and complicated planning may not be necessary.

A radiation plan can be broken down into two key aspects: (1) the dose and number of fractions of radiation prescribed to the cancer (the *target*); and (2) the dose prescribed to the normal structures.

1. The Target

The radiation plan will include a target that has been drawn by the radiation oncologist. This is almost always referred to as the *planning target volume*, or PTV. The PTV is a structure that includes the places where the cancer is known to be (that is, the tumor itself and lymph nodes known to have cancer in them) and places where the cancer might spread (usually lymph nodes in the area), and it incorporates a small safety margin for positioning uncertainties or movement.

Figure 7 shows a CT simulation scan for a man with prostate cancer (you can view a color version of this figure at http://quality cancertreatment.com/links). On the left, we see the normal organs outlined, including the *femurs* (F), which are the hip bones, the bladder (B), and the rectum (R). We also see the target: the prostate (P) and organs right behind, the *seminal vesicles* (SV), where the cancer can spread. Around those, with a slight margin for error, is the PTV. On the right is the radiation plan. The area getting the prescription dose (which is 76 Gy) or more is indicated by the innermost outline. As we move outward from that 76 Gy outline, each line that we come to signifies an area receiving a lower dose. The lines that you see include 50 percent (38 Gy) and 25 percent (19 Gy) of the prescription dose. You can see that the highest-dose region in the right-hand picture corresponds very well with the target in the left-hand picture.*

---

* In your own radiation plan, you might also see some structures *within* the PTV. These may include the *gross tumor volume* (GTV) and the *clinical target volume* (CTV). The GTV indicates where the doctor can see cancer on the scan. In figure 7, we can't see the cancer within the prostate, so there is no GTV. The CTV indicates where the cancer might be—it includes the GTV with margin for spread, and it sometimes includes some other areas at risk of harboring cancer. On the left side of the figure above, the CTV includes the prostate and an area just behind it, the seminal vesicles, outlined by the inner octopus-type shape right above the circular prostate. From the CTV, the doctor adds another safety margin for motion or setup uncertainties to make the PTV.

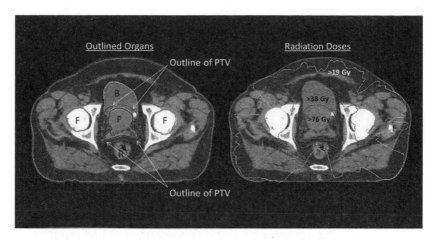

Figure 7. Radiation Plan for Treatment of Prostate Cancer

Go over these questions with your doctor:

- *Can you show me the planning target volume in my radiation plan?*

- *Have all the places where cancer is known been included (that is, the primary tumor and any lymph nodes with cancer)?*

- *Is the planning target volume getting a sufficient dose?*

  - Usually, we try to make sure that 95 percent of the planning target volume receives 95 percent of the dose. So if the doctor has prescribed a dose of 60 Gy in 30 fractions, nearly all of the PTV should be receiving 57 Gy (95 percent of 60 Gy).

2. The Normal Tissues

In a radiation plan, the normal tissues of the body are usually called *organs at risk*, or OARs. For a patient with prostate cancer, the

OARs include the rectum, the bladder, the femurs, and a few other structures. For a patient with lung cancer, they include the normal lung tissues, the heart, major blood vessels, major airways, the chest wall and ribs, and the esophagus.

The radiation plan will minimize the dose of radiation being delivered to OARs, but they will receive some amount of radiation. The goal is to keep this amount as low as possible while making sure the tumor receives a sufficient radiation dose.

Your radiation plan should include a list of all the structures in the radiation plan (including the normal tissues), along with the doses that those structures will be receiving. A simplified version is shown in table 5.

Table 5. Doses to Normal Organs in a Sample Prostate Cancer Radiation Plan

Organ	Maximum Dose	Average Dose
Bladder	78.3 Gy	48.4 Gy
Left Femur	42.1 Gy	16.5 Gy
Rectum	78.5 Gy	35.6 Gy
Right Femur	41.0 Gy	16.3 Gy

The list tells your doctor that some areas of the bladder and rectum are receiving very high doses of radiation; this is necessary because they are right up against the target or sometimes within the target itself. The bones are getting more modest doses of radiation.

How much radiation is safe? There is no hard cutoff for any organ. We just know that as the dose increases, the probability of most types of complications increases. Doctors have a list of doses that they try not to exceed for certain organs—these are called *tolerance doses*. We usually set the tolerance dose at a level that will produce no more than a 5 percent risk of serious complications to that organ within five years. In some circumstances, the tolerance doses will be exceeded somewhat if there is no alternative. As we discussed in chapter 7, all the risks must be considered in the context of the potential benefits, and sometimes the chance to cure a potentially lethal cancer involves risks. The plan that I showed you above would be considered safe, although there is a small risk of serious side effects to any of the OARs.

Ask your doctor:

- *Have all the organs at risk in the area been outlined?*

- *Are there any organs at risk that are receiving a dose that exceeds their tolerance?*

- *What are my risks of complications with the doses that are being delivered to the normal tissues?*

If you have received radiation in the past, make sure your doctor is aware of the radiation dose and has obtained a copy of your old radiation records. The doses previously delivered to your normal tissues will need to be taken into account in your new radiation plan.

Designing radiation plans for palliative treatments may not require the same level of complexity, because the radiation doses are usually much lower and the chances of side effects are usually smaller. Also, when treating palliatively, time is usually of the essence: if a patient is having substantial pain, it is usually preferable to start a simple radiation plan immediately rather than taking many days to design a more complicated plan that might not be any better at improving symptoms. For a palliative radiation plan, the doctor may not even need to outline any targets, but just to design a beam or two of radiation that includes the area in question. However, you can still ask your doctor to show you a copy of the radiation treatment plan that has been designed for you.

During Radiation

The radiation therapists will position you and deliver each radiation fraction. They should take the time to explain what they are doing at each step of the way. They are normally happy to answer questions and are very knowledgeable about radiation treatments and the experiences of other patients undergoing treatments like yours.

You will usually meet with your radiation doctor weekly, or every two weeks, during the radiation. These visits are mostly to check you for side effects and to help you manage any symptoms that arise. The side effects are usually related to the area being treated (apart from fatigue). For the prostate cancer patient above, side effects to the rectum, bladder, and skin would be most likely. For the head and neck cancer patient earlier in this chapter, we would be worried about issues with pain and swallowing and taste, which can lead to weight loss and dehydration. Give your doctor an honest summary of your symptoms, and ask if anything can be done to make them better.

You can also ask your doctor if there are any issues with your day-to-day positioning for radiation. These visits are also a good time to ask any lingering questions about your treatment and about next steps after treatment (which we discuss in chapter 13).

Wrap-up and Mini-checklist

After reading this chapter, radiation treatment should no longer be mysterious to you. You've learned how radiation is designed and that numerous checks have to be in place to make sure things are done safely. Safety can be achieved only when the system is geared toward double- and triple-checking.

Here is a list of the main questions to ask your radiation team:

☐ *Even though you are recommending radiation, are there any other alternative treatments available (like surgery)?*

If the answer is yes, then you should ask:

- *How do you know that radiation is better than these other options?*

- *Can I meet with those specialists (for example, a surgeon) to discuss those alternatives?*

☐ *Will I need other treatments during radiation (like chemotherapy) or after (like chemotherapy or surgery)?*

If the answer is yes, then ask:

- *What is the added benefit of radiation over just having these other treatments?*

☐ *What is the dose and fractionation of radiation that you are prescribing, and is it standard for this situation?*

☐ *Can my treatment be delivered in a smaller number of fractions and still have the same effect, without more side effects?*

☐ *For my type of cancer, are you considered a high-volume radiation center and a high-volume radiation oncologist?*

☐ *Does your center meet the quality assurance requirements from recognized professional organizations like the American Association of Physicists in Medicine and the American Society for Radiation Oncology?*

- In countries outside the United States, other similar guidelines might be used.

☐ *Will my radiation plan be double-checked by a second doctor?*

☐ *Who else double-checks my radiation plan after it's done?*

☐ *Can you review my radiation plan with me?*

☐ *How well am I being positioned during my radiation, and how is this monitored?*

CHAPTER 11

Systemic Therapy: More Than Just a Drip

Systemic therapies—drugs that are given by mouth or by injection that circulate throughout the body—have been a major contributor to our success against cancer. Because these drugs enter the bloodstream, they can potentially attack cancer cells anywhere in the body. Their ability to circulate widely differs from surgery and radiation, which are essentially local therapies, acting only where they are directed.*

Chemotherapy is the most common type of systemic therapy. Although the word "chemotherapy" originally described drugs that were used to treat infectious diseases, it now refers to many of the drugs that are used to treat cancer. Early uses of chemotherapy were very crude (including nitrogen mustard to treat lymphoma in the Second World War, which we no longer use), but chemotherapy is now much more sophisticated. We have had enormous improvements, both in terms of the drugs used to treat cancer and the drugs used to prevent and reduce side effects.[92]

---

* As mentioned in chapter 2, there is one rare exception to this rule with radiation: the abscopal effect.

The other major types of systemic therapy include *hormone therapies* (which block the hormones that some cancers need in order to grow, often used for breast and prostate cancers), *targeted therapies* (drugs that are designed to attack a specific target on a cancer cell, used in several types of cancers, including breast, colon, lung, and prostate), and *immunotherapies* (drugs that allow the immune system to better detect and attack cancer cells).

If systemic therapy is an option for your type of cancer, this chapter is going to help you decide if it is right for you and will teach you how to double-check the treatment recommended for you. Many patient information books provide the basic questions about chemotherapy, such as "Why do I need it?" "Which drugs will I receive?" "How is it given?" and "What is the treatment schedule?" In this chapter, I will assume you've already read the standard patient information material; if you haven't, please read the chapter 8 resources first to see where to find it. The goal of this chapter is to go beyond those questions to help you receive high-quality systemic therapy.

Goals of Systemic Therapy

There are several reasons why we use systemic therapy in cancer treatment, and each reason is given a different medical term. These terms are important for you to learn so you can understand the benefits of chemotherapy in your situation and be able to double-check the chemotherapy drugs and doses that are being used.

In some uncommon cases, the goal of systemic therapy is curative—to try to eradicate a cancer. Currently, chemotherapy can be given with curative intent for only a small number of cancers, such as leukemias and lymphomas and for testicular cancer that is metastatic.[93]

More commonly, systemic therapy is considered a helper, meant to kill any microscopic cancer cells that might be hiding somewhere in the body after surgery or radiation.* For example, many women with breast cancer often undergo surgery first, to remove all the known cancer in the breast and armpit, sometimes followed by radiation to those areas. Afterward, even though there may be no visible cancer left, systemic therapy is often warranted (given as chemotherapy and/or hormone therapy) in case there are microscopic cells left behind in the breast, armpit, or elsewhere in the body. This systemic therapy can substantially improve the chances of cure.[94] In this situation, when systemic therapy is given "in addition to" the main treatment, we call it *adjuvant therapy*, which is defined as extra cancer treatment that is given *after* the main treatment in order to reduce the risk of the cancer coming back. If the order of treatments is reversed and systemic therapy is given *before* the main treatment, we use the terms *neoadjuvant therapy* or *induction therapy*.

In other situations, systemic therapy is given during radiation treatment to try to make the radiation work better. Patients with lung cancer, head and neck cancer, esophageal cancer, and many other types of cancers will receive chemotherapy and radiation together to improve the chances of cure, and in this case, we use the term *concurrent* to describe the timing of the chemotherapy.[95]

Finally, in a situation where a cancer cannot be cured, palliative systemic therapy can be used to try to extend life and/or improve quality of life, by reducing the burden of cancer while not eradicating it completely.

Check the Benefits

In chapter 7, I wrote about how to weigh the risks and benefits of any treatment, and those considerations apply here. If you haven't already

---

* I specify "microscopic" because systemic therapy usually doesn't kill large clumps of cancer cells; that's why it is usually not able to cure metastatic cancers. Recall from chapter 2 that no scan can detect microscopic spots of cancer.

read through that chapter, then take some time to do so now. The key message in that chapter is that the benefits of treatment need to outweigh the risks.

For patients receiving systemic therapy, you should be able to get a very precise estimate of the benefits. For example, if chemotherapy is an option, you can get information about exactly how much of a benefit the chemotherapy will provide. Some of the resources that can provide this information are listed at the end of this chapter.

Check the Drugs and Doses

Different systemic therapy drugs work for different types of cancers. A drug that is useful for lung cancer might not be active against breast cancer or prostate cancer. It's worth checking to make sure that the drug and dosage of the systemic therapy that your doctor is prescribing are correct for your situation.

There are two good resources to help you assess the drugs and doses for your type of cancer. The first is the NCCN's physician guidelines (described in chapter 8), which often list preferred chemotherapy regimens. The second is the list of chemotherapy protocols published by the BC Cancer Agency (BCCA), discussed in more detail at the end of this chapter.

There are several important things to keep in mind about systemic therapy dosing. First, different cancer drugs are dosed in different ways. For some drugs, it's a standard dose given to essentially all patients (for instance, 20 mg of tamoxifen for breast cancer patients). For other drugs, it's based on your weight and height; and for some others, it's based on the measurements of how well your kidneys work or other parameters. Ask your doctor how your dose will be calculated and ensure that your accurate weight and height are on file.* I have seen errors in chemotherapy delivery where the wrong dose was given because the patient's weight was entered incorrectly.

Second, different institutions may use slightly different chemotherapy protocols for the same type of cancer. There is often a major component of physician judgment in selecting chemotherapy, particularly when there are several effective drugs that differ in side effects. Ask your doctor if the regimen prescribed for you matches one of the regimens in the guidelines, and if not, ask him why there is a difference.

Third, doctors may lower the doses of some drugs based on an individual patient's specific situation, particularly if the patient is frail or has other medical issues, such as kidney or heart problems. Ask your doctor if these factors have been taken into account when prescribing your treatment.

Side Effects and Management

Side effects from systemic therapy vary enormously, based on the type of drug being prescribed, the dose, and the individual patient. For some side effects, it might be critical to seek medical attention even if they seem very mild (for example, a slight fever can be a serious concern if you've received chemotherapy that reduces your white blood cell count). Other side effects are of no concern if they are mild, but they can become life-threatening if severe (such as diarrhea).

If you are having side effects that your doctors are having trouble getting under control, it might be helpful to check the guidelines for management of those symptoms. Sometimes the guidelines will

---

*   For drugs that are dosed based on height and weight, your doctor often calculates your *body surface area* (BSA) to determine the dose. You can double-check your BSA at http://www.medcalc.com/body.html.

suggest an approach that your doctor may not have considered. Guidelines are available to help address such issues as nausea, fatigue, diarrhea, constipation, pain, drug-induced rashes, and hot flashes.*

For some side effects that are troublesome or threaten to cause problems (such as low blood counts), your doctor may consider a reduction in dose, or a delay, in your next cycle. (See the list of questions at the end of this chapter for some specific things to ask your doctor regarding side effects from systemic therapy.)

Keep a List of Treatments

It's helpful to keep a record of the systemic therapies that you receive. These records become important if you ever need systemic therapy again (either for the same cancer or a new one), since some drugs have lifetime dose limits. The records are also useful for patients who develop treatment-related side effects in the future, as the doctors may want records of which treatments were delivered previously. If your treatment information is needed in the future, your new doctors can usually contact your previous hospital to get that information, but this can lead to unnecessary delays. The cancer care spreadsheet in the Patient Toolkit (http://www.qualitycancertreatment.com/toolkit) contains a tab where you can input data on the treatments you've received, including systemic therapies.

Choosing a Treatment Center

In the previous two chapters on surgery and radiation, we learned that practice makes perfect: surgeons who do a particular operation

---

* See, for example, Cancer.Net's "Side Effects" web page and the BC Cancer Agency's "Symptom & Side Effect Management Resource Guide" web page, both linked at http://www.qualitycancertreatment.com/a08.

more frequently tend to obtain better outcomes, as do radiation oncologists who treat a certain cancer more frequently.

The relationship between systemic therapy volumes and outcomes is not as well studied and can be difficult to tease out. For example, a patient who has surgery at a high-volume center would often also have her chemotherapy there, so she'd receive both treatments at a high-volume institution. The better outcomes that we see at high-volume surgical and radiation centers probably reflect some benefit to being a high-volume chemotherapy center as well. In the few studies that look at the relationship between hospital volumes and outcomes for patients who are receiving only chemotherapy (without surgery or radiation), similar patterns emerge. In one study of patients receiving palliative chemotherapy for pancreatic cancer, those treated at a high-volume center had a 10 percent higher chance of being alive one year after diagnosis compared with patients treated at low-volume centers.[96] In another study of patients receiving chemotherapy for *acute myeloid leukemia*, a blood cancer, patients treated at high-volume centers had a mortality rate of 2 percent, compared with 5 percent at low-volume centers.[97]

Even though the data is weaker for chemotherapy, it's worth asking your medical oncologist how many patients per year with your diagnosis receive chemotherapy at his hospital and in his individual practice. If the number sounds low, it's worth discussing the potential value of a high-volume center. In some instances, larger centers may have arrangements with community hospitals to deliver treatments closer to home. In this case, ask how your treatment will be monitored and what safety checks are in place to ensure that your chemotherapy is being delivered safely and according to plan.

Wrap-up and Mini-checklist

In this chapter, we've learned that systemic therapy is a key component of cancer treatment. With systemic therapy, it is often possible to get a precise estimate of the potential benefits, to make better-informed decisions. You can also double-check that the drugs and doses delivered are correct.

Here is a list of some of the key questions to ask your medical oncologist:

- *What are the goals of systemic therapy in my situation?*

- *What are the specific benefits in my case? What are my predicted outcomes with or without systemic therapy?*

- *Do you commonly treat patients with my type of cancer?*

- *Which drugs will you be using? Are these consistent with guidelines?*

- *Can you or a team member show me the numbers you've used to calculate the dose, such as my weight or kidney function?*

- *Which side effects should I be most concerned about?*

- *Are there medications I need to take preventively to avoid side effects or medications I need on hand in case side effects develop?*

- *When should I seek medical attention? If I need medical attention, can I reach you or another on-call medical oncologist, or do I need to go to the emergency room? Will the doctors I see have access to all of my treatment records?*

Resources

Calculating the Benefits of Systemic Therapy

A few online calculators are available that can provide an estimate of the benefits of systemic therapy. If there is a calculator available for your type of cancer, sit down with your doctor and review the results. Keep in mind that the calculators aren't perfect, but it's fair to rely on them to give ballpark estimates, usually within a few percentage points.[98] Sometimes these calculators are unavailable for periods of time as they update their formulas based on the latest information.

For women with breast cancer, the PREDICT tool (http://www.predict.nhs.uk) allows you to enter some of the parameters from your pathology report, along with a few more pieces of information (such as your age), and in return, it provides the following information: the percentage of women who would be alive without any adjuvant therapy at 5 and 10 years, and the additional percentage who would be alive at those times by adding in hormonal treatment, chemotherapy, and targeted therapy, if applicable.

Adjuvant! Online (https://adjuvantonline.com) provides similar calculators to estimate the benefits of chemotherapy for breast, lung, colon, and other cancers. The Adjuvant! Online website stipulates that it is for use only by physicians, so ask your doctor to sit down with you and use it at one of your visits. Some doctors do this already and print out the reports for their patients.

If there is no calculator available for your type of cancer, your oncologist may be able to direct you to one and help you find that information. You can also find out about the specific benefits of chemotherapy using the resources at the end of chapter 8 (such as UpToDate or the NCCN Guidelines). They might tell you, for example, that the addition of drug X after surgery provides a

10 percent increase in survival after five years. Ask your doctor specifically about the numbers for your situation.

Checking the Drugs and Doses

As mentioned earlier in the chapter, two good resources for checking on your dosing are the NCCN's physician guidelines and the BCCA's "Chemotherapy Protocols" web page.* The BCCA protocols cover many of the common drug regimens used for many types of cancer. They are organized by type of cancer (lung, breast, prostate, and so forth), the goal of treatment (for example, adjuvant or palliative), and the specific drugs used. The protocols specify the doses of the drugs, additional medications to be given with them (to prevent nausea, for instance), and some of the other safety checks that should be in place (like checking blood counts on the day of treatment). You can print these out and bring them to your own medical oncologist to discuss.

---

* Linked at http://www.qualitycancertreatment.com/a08.

CHAPTER 12

Clinical Trials: Sometimes a Better Option

When doctors have an idea for a new intervention to improve cancer treatment, they will test it in patients by doing a clinical trial. Clinical trials have allowed medicine to move forward, and as a result, patients who are diagnosed with cancer today benefit because of patients who joined clinical trials in the past. But patients who are diagnosed with cancer today might also benefit from joining a clinical trial themselves.

Clinical trials can test a wide variety of things. Often the goal of the trial is to try to improve cure rates by testing new drugs, new combinations of drugs, or new approaches to radiation or surgery. In other cases, the goal of the trial is to improve quality of life by using treatments that might be less toxic. In some cases, clinical trials don't evaluate cancer treatments at all, but study things like patient education, counseling, lifestyle interventions (such as exercise, weight loss, dietary changes, yoga), or different approaches to patient decision making.

Only a small minority of patients—fewer than 1 in 10 patients—enroll in a clinical trial. Many times, the reason for this low enrollment is that patients simply are not offered the opportunity to join a trial.[99] Yet the National Comprehensive Cancer Network, the group responsible for many of the guidelines we've discussed, clearly states: "NCCN believes that the best management for any cancer patient is in a clinical trial."[100]

In this chapter, we'll discuss the types of clinical trials and why it's important to consider joining a clinical trial. I will provide some tips on how to find one specific to your type of cancer.

Types of Clinical Trials

When considering joining a clinical trial, it's important to be aware of the goal of the trial. If you are looking for a trial that might increase your chances of cure but mistakenly join one that is looking at safety of a new compound, then you are not necessarily furthering your goals.

When testing new drugs or new approaches, researchers tend to classify trials into categories or *phases*. A *phase I trial* is when doctors test a new treatment (usually a new drug), mostly to assess the safety and side effects of the treatment. A phase I trial is usually not meant to check if the treatment actually works. Many patients who join phase I trials are not aware of this distinction; they believe that the goal of the phase I trial is to try to cure their cancer or to see if the drug works.[101]

In some phase I trials, patients do get lucky, and the drug being assessed for safety turns out to be highly active in their type of cancer. For example, in 2009, a phase I study was launched to test a new immunotherapy drug, called nivolumab, for patients with stage IV melanoma. The trial was designed to assess the safety and optimum dose levels. It turned out that nivolumab was highly active in melanoma and years later became a proven treatment once larger randomized studies were done.[102] But some of the patients who entered the original phase I trial did very well and achieved long-term remission after getting the drug.[103]

If a treatment appears to be safe in a phase I trial, then a *phase II trial* is usually the next step, in which the treatment is given to a larger group of people. The main goal of the phase II trial is to get an initial indication about the effectiveness of the treatment. Often all the patients who join the phase II trial receive the new treatment, but sometimes the phase II trial can be a randomized trial, wherein different patients will receive different treatments, to allow for an initial comparison between groups.*

If the treatment appears to be promising in a phase II trial, then a definitive study is done, a *phase III trial.* The goal of a phase III trial is to make a final comparison to see if the new treatment is better than, or as good as, currently available treatments. Phase III trials are randomized, usually involving hundreds of patients at several institutions.

Sometimes trials differ slightly in their goals and design from this general paradigm, and there are other phases (including phase 0 and phase IV) that can be used in some specific situations.

Joining a Clinical Trial Can Be Beneficial

The main reason for joining a clinical trial is to improve cancer care for future patients. But you might also be able to improve your own chances by entering a trial. There are a few ways that entering a trial could provide benefits.

First, entering a trial might get you access to a new treatment that would not be available otherwise. If that treatment works, then you benefit. Besides the immunotherapy example above, there are numerous other examples of patients getting new experimental drugs that prove to be helpful.[104] However, there are no guarantees—

---

*   For more details about randomization and why we use it, see chapter 5. If you wish to learn more about the different types of clinical trials, see https://www.nccn.org/patients/resources/clinical_trials/phases.aspx.

sometimes the new drug is not helpful at all, or even harmful. But in principle, trials are launched because researchers believe that the new treatment will be an improvement over what is currently available.

Second, even if the new treatment itself is not helpful, the overall process of being in a trial might be helpful. There are a few reasons why you might get better quality of care when in a trial:

1. Institutions that run clinical trials might be more organized and provide better care. In some branches of medicine, institutions that run clinical trials appear to have better outcomes than institutions that don't run trials.[105]

2. Trials provide a road map for you. Your road map will provide you with a list of your appointments, tests, and treatment, so you will clearly know what is required at what time.

3. Your doctor also gets a road map, one that includes specific directions on how to deliver the treatment on a trial. For example, a trial involving radiation and chemotherapy will usually tell the doctors exactly which areas to treat with radiation, exactly which dose of radiation to deliver, which chemotherapy drugs to deliver, which doses to use, and how to manage side effects.

4. Sometimes there is more peer review for patients who are entered in trials. Some trials mandate that patients must be discussed by the multidisciplinary team (discussed in chapter 8) before enrollment, whereas others include a review of radiation plans, imaging, or pathology.

5. Finally, some patients find that they get an additional personal touch by being in a clinical trial. Often there is a study nurse or a research coordinator who can act as your point of contact for any issues that arise. This person can make sure

that all the tests, scans, and appointments are being done on time and not missed, and your point of contact will also help to make sure that the trial protocol is followed.*

Although there are several good reasons for joining a trial, we don't have data that conclusively proves that these benefits translate into longer survival. Some studies are promising. One large study of over 500,000 patients in California found that those who enrolled in trials had a lower risk of death than patients not treated in trials.[106] Another large study also suggested that there is a benefit in survival for patients entering trials but that these benefits are mostly restricted to cancers for which the prognosis is not very good, such as lung, pancreas, and brain cancer.[107] However, other smaller studies have not shown a benefit. Reassuringly, none have shown that patients who participated in trials did worse overall.[108]

So although the survival benefit of entering a trial has not been conclusively proven, it may exist. And when you add that to all the other possible benefits—accessing new treatments, getting a road map for you and your doctors, better contact with your team, and importantly, the possibility of improving cancer treatment for future patients—it's worth considering entering a trial.

How to Find Clinical Trials

There are several ways to find clinical trials that might be applicable to you:

1. Ask your doctors. Tell them you are interested in a clinical trial, and they will be able to tell you if any are available. If

---

* To read more about how clinical trials can provide structure and a personal touch that patients appreciate, see http://www.qualitycancertreatment.com/blog/clinicaltrials.

they have none, then ask them if they know of any promising trials at other centers that you could access.

2. Check the clinical trial directories. There are several online searchable directories that list clinical trials (some of which are listed at the end of this chapter).

3. Try the National Cancer Institute. The NCI is the US government's main institution for cancer research and is considered a world leader in cancer research. Patients who participate in trials at the NCI have their medical costs covered. International patients may also participate. (To read more about NCI trials, go to http://www.cancer.gov and type "clinical trials" into the search box.)

4. Call other institutions. If there are other cancer institutions in your area, or high-quality centers that you'd consider traveling to, call their patient intake line and ask. Just tell them your situation and ask if there are trials available. You might say, "Hi, I'm a patient with stage III breast cancer, and I'm looking for clinical trials—do you have any that might suit me?"

If you find a trial using one of these methods, you will have to ask about the associated costs of the trial. In some cases, participation will be free, but in other cases, there may be a cost, particularly in an insurance-based system if the hospital is out-of-network. The institution running the trials may have some ways to offset some of the costs.

Wrap-up and Mini-checklist

In this chapter, we learned that only a small minority of cancer patients enroll in a clinical trial. There are several types of clinical trials, including phase I trials, which assess safety; phase II trials, which give an early idea of the effectiveness; and phase III trials, which provide a definitive comparison of a new intervention versus standard treatment. The main reason to join a clinical trial is that it may be helpful for patients in the future. However, some research suggests that there may be benefits even for the patients who join the trials.

Here is a list of questions to ask your medical team:

- *Do you have any clinical trials available for me? If not, do you have any suggestions for trials I can pursue at other centers?*

- *What is the goal of the clinical trial you are offering to me?*

  - If the goal of the trial is to evaluate a new drug, ask: *Is there already some data to suggest that this drug might be helpful for my type of cancer?*

- *Can you explain the trial to me and what treatment(s) are delivered?*

- *What are the potential risks and benefits of participating?*

- *Does this trial require any special tests or procedures?*

  - Some trials require extra scans, blood tests, biopsies, or other procedures.

- *Are there costs associated with joining this trial?*

Resources

Clinical Trial Directories

Clinical trial directories require a bit of knowledge of medical lingo, so you'll need to make sure you understand your diagnosis and stage, and you may also need to use a medical dictionary. For help on how to use the directories, see the "Finding Clinical Trials" video in the online Patient Toolkit (http://www.qualitycancertreatment.com /toolkit).

- For patients in the United States and elsewhere, start with https://www.clinicaltrials.gov. This is a comprehensive list of trials, mainly from the United States, but also from other countries.

- In Canada: http://www.canadiancancertrials.ca.

- In Europe: https://www.clinicaltrialsregister.eu.

- In Australia: http://www.australiancancertrials.gov.au.

Review your search with your medical team. They can help you determine which trials are most applicable and also facilitate referrals, if necessary. Most of these trial directories include a contact person for each study, and you can also e-mail them directly for more information.

CHAPTER 13

After Treatment Is Finished

The end of cancer treatment—finishing chemotherapy, radiation, and/or surgery—signifies a big change. During treatment, patients are kept busy, attending appointments and focusing on getting through treatment and managing side effects.

The end of treatment is looked forward to as something to be celebrated. At our cancer center, the radiation department has an enormous, loud gong that patients strike with a hammer once they've completed their radiation. Shortly after it was installed, having been donated by a local business, one of my patients noticed that there was no equivalent noisemaker for patients completing chemotherapy. She donated a large bell for that purpose. Now our department is a cacophony of sound. Obviously, the end of treatment is worth celebrating.

But the end of treatment can also be a big letdown. The frequent visits are replaced by infrequent checkups. The busy schedule eases off. Patients have more time to think about whether the cancer is cured and about their side effects. There may be concerns about physical appearance, uncertainty about their future health, or anger about the toll that cancer has taken on their lives.

This part of the cancer journey, after treatment is finished, can be incredibly difficult, as patients may feel like they are no longer actively treating their cancer but just waiting with their fingers crossed. Having a road map for the future and an understanding of what's to come, and what needs to be done, can help alleviate these concerns.

Historically, *survivorship*—the time after cancer treatment—has been about detecting whether the cancer has come back and sometimes also helping to deal with side effects. Until recently, there was little focus on emotional, financial, or mental health.

Patients have historically been passive participants in the survivorship process, coming to appointments and having tests done as recommended by their doctors, without much of an idea of the overall long-term plan or goals. Yet missed appointments, missed scans, or unmet emotional needs can have an impact on survival and quality of life.

In this chapter, you are going to learn how to take an active role in your survivorship and how to make sure that all the correct tests and visits are arranged and that your physical and emotional needs are being met. These interventions can help improve your quality of care, detect recurrences if the cancer comes back, and give you confidence that your needs will be fulfilled.

The Importance of Follow-up

Audie Harold was a 42-year-old mother of two when she was diagnosed with colon cancer. She had been feeling tired, and her blood counts were low and not improving with iron replacement. Her doctor referred her for a colonoscopy, where a camera was inserted into her rectum and snaked backward through her large intestine. A tumor was found, and a biopsy revealed colon cancer.

She was treated with surgery and adjuvant chemotherapy. Her scans and blood tests after treatment showed no evidence of cancer, so she settled into a regular routine of follow-up appointments. Her surgeon's office would call her to schedule each one. When she didn't receive a call after her 18-month visit, she assumed that her surgeon didn't need to see her. She had other things on her mind: she and her husband were planning an extended getaway with the kids, spending a year overseas as a way to reboot after a difficult time.

About two weeks before it was time to leave, one of her friends asked her if she had arranged for follow-up for her colon cancer in her new location. "No," Audie replied. "I haven't seen my surgeon in several months, and I didn't realize I needed any more follow-up." So she contacted her doctors and asked.

Sure enough, ongoing follow-up was needed, and her next appointment was due right away. Her surgeon scrambled to arrange a CT scan, and the news was disappointing: the cancer had returned.

There was reason for a bit of optimism: the cancer had returned in only a few locations, and it had been caught early enough that it could be removed, with the goal of cure.

But it was almost a missed opportunity. She hadn't been made aware of the need for follow-up, and her appointments had almost fallen through the cracks. If she had left on her trip, it may have been several months until the cancer was detected, and the possibility of cure might have been lost.

Your Personalized Follow-up Plan

Follow-up visits have several important purposes. The traditional goals of follow-up have been to determine whether a cancer has come back and to manage any ongoing complications from treatment. But medicine has evolved, and appropriate follow-up care nowadays is more complex; it includes efforts to detect or prevent additional cancers or side effects, as well as assessment of any ongoing psychological, emotional, and social issues (or any other health needs) that can be addressed.[109]

Each type of cancer has specific guidelines around the necessary follow-up procedures required. For some cancers, close follow-up and regular imaging are required, whereas for others, the follow-up is more spread out, imaging may not be necessary, and the follow-up might be done by someone other than your oncologist. Proper follow-up is a balance: too few visits or investigations can lead to undetected problems, but too many can lead to wasted time and money, unnecessary anxiety, and, in the case of extra scans, unnecessary radiation exposure.

A major effort is under way to standardize follow-up care and keep patients from falling through the cracks by using the *survivorship care plan* (SCP) tool, which is recommended by the US Institute of Medicine and several other organizations. An SCP is a document made up of two sections: first, a summary of the treatment; and second, an outline of the plan for ongoing follow-up.[110] A detailed outline of the components of SCPs, along with where to find one for your type of cancer, is provided at the end of this chapter.

Cancer programs have not been using SCPs consistently, even though they were recommended more than a decade ago. One study done in 2014 looked at 36 different cancer programs to see how many of those programs were successfully using SCPs. The study defined three benchmarks for success: creating SCPs for 75 percent of patients, delivering them to 75 percent of patients, and also delivering copies to 75 percent of family doctors or primary care providers. Of the 36 programs studied, only one met all three criteria.[111]

But the numbers are about to improve. Not only are patients going to become more aware of SCPs, but they will soon be required for many institutions. The Commission on Cancer is an organization aimed at improving outcomes for cancer patients by setting standards for cancer programs, and programs that meet those standards can become designated as CoC-accredited. There are approximately

1,500 accredited centers in the United States. The CoC will require that by the end of 2018, at least 75 percent of eligible patients are to receive SCPs at a given cancer treatment facility for it to be accredited.[112] So it is expected that the use of SCPs is going to increase rapidly.

We don't yet have data to show that SCPs improve outcomes for cancer patients. Very few randomized trials exist. Among the examples of randomized trials that have been done, the studies have looked at short-term outcomes in women with breast cancer or endometrial cancer who tended to have early-stage disease. The studies didn't find any benefits in those populations.[113] But these studies don't provide definitive answers that apply to other types of cancer. The benefits of SCPs are more likely to be shown in patient groups who have a high risk of recurrence; in the low-risk groups thus far studied, for which the chance of cure is already very high, SCPs are unlikely to improve cancer outcomes that much because a large majority of the patients are already cured. Other randomized trials are ongoing.

In the meantime, not everyone believes that randomized trials are needed to prove the benefits of SCPs. In commenting on the lack of randomized trials for SCPs, Thomas Smith and Claire Snyder of Johns Hopkins pose this question: "Perhaps there is a role for common sense in medicine; if something is simple, cheap, and not harmful, if it gets all patients to a level playing field and can be updated, how much proof do we need?"[114]

It's worth considering getting an SCP. If you are not offered one, you can find one online using the resources at the end of this chapter and print it out to review with your doctor, or you can ask your doctor to provide one for you.

Checking the Recommendations

Once you've filled out the SCP with your doctor, you can check your plan against published guidelines. The NCCN physician guidelines (see chapter 8) usually have a section on follow-up, which is also called "surveillance" or "survivorship" in the documents. After treatment of colon cancer, like Audie had, the recommendation is for: (1) a visit (including history and physical) with a CEA (a special blood test) every 3–6 months in the first two years, then less frequently thereafter; (2) CT scanning every 6–12 months after treatment; and (3) colonoscopy at regular intervals. This differs from breast cancer, for which the frequency of visits is different, there are no CT scans (just annual mammograms), and no regular blood tests.

You can double-check the recommendations in your SCP against the NCCN guidelines for follow-up for your type and stage of cancer, and if there are discrepancies, ask your doctor about them.

Attitude and Mood

Depression is common in patients with cancer. Approximately 10–20 percent of cancer patients develop depression at some point in their journey, either at diagnosis, during treatment, or afterward.[115] This is much higher than in the general population, where the rate of depression is around 4 percent.[116] Historically, mood issues have been an afterthought for oncologists, who were usually focused first on treating the cancer itself, and then on managing side effects.

We now realize that depression is a major issue and can have important consequences. Patients who are depressed have worse outcomes, both in terms of survival from the cancer and complications from treatment.[117] Cancer patients who are depressed are more likely to visit their non–mental-health-care providers, visit the emergency room, be admitted to the hospital, or be readmitted to the hospital within 30 days of a previous admission, compared with cancer patients without depression.[118]

These findings resulted from studies that compared depressed patients with nondepressed patients. When you look at the other end of the spectrum—patients with an especially positive attitude—it's often suggested by survivors and some health care practitioners that a "fighting spirit" can help improve outcomes against cancers. This does not appear to be the case.[119]

The mechanisms of the relationship between depression and cancer survival are unclear. Three main theories have been proposed. First, it may be that hormones related to stress, depression, or anxiety are to blame, as some of these hormones (such as cortisol) can impair immune function. Second, depressed patients may be less likely to adhere to treatment recommendations. Third, some of the symptoms of advanced cancer are similar to symptoms of depression (including sleep disturbance, fatigue, and difficulty concentrating, which we will discuss below), so the diagnosis of depression may just reflect more advanced underlying cancer.[120]

Regardless of the mechanisms, doctors and patients should be aware of the risk of depression. The symptoms of depression can include not only a depressed mood, but also a loss of interest or pleasure in most activities; changes in weight, appetite, sleep, or activity; fatigue; difficulty concentrating; and feelings of guilt or worthlessness. Sometimes there are associated thoughts of self-harm.

If you have feelings that may be related to depression, talk to your oncologist immediately.* Even if your mood is good, it's worth asking where to turn if you do develop emotional distress or depressive symptoms.

---

* Also see http://www.cancer.net/coping-with-cancer/managing-emotions.

Cigarettes and Tobacco

Continued smoking after a diagnosis of cancer is associated with several bad outcomes. In general, patients who continue to smoke have higher risks of treatment-related complications, cancer relapse, and the development of new cancers, and they tend to have a shorter overall survival.[121]

Doctors have overlooked the importance of smoking cessation. As a profession, we haven't done a good job of helping patients: although we often ask about smoking and advise patients to quit, we usually don't take the important next steps. These include assessing whether a patient wants to quit, assisting them in quitting (often with counseling and/or medications), and arranging follow-up on the issue.[122] As a result, our patients often don't get the proper support that can dramatically increase the chances of quitting.

If you are a smoker, ask your doctor for assistance in quitting and to follow your progress during the quitting process. At some cancer centers, there will be a smoking cessation program that you can access.

Weight Loss and Dietary Changes

Will interventions like weight loss and changes in your diet help to keep cancer away? For most cancers, the answer is no. Although being overweight can increase the risk of recurrence for some cancers, trials of interventions where patients have been instructed to lose weight or make dietary changes have not been overly encouraging. We will discuss some of these interventions, such as a low-fat diet, in chapter 15.

Sometimes the relationship between dietary intake and outcomes can be complex. Recommendations around alcohol consumption are a good example of this. Reducing alcohol consumption is important if you have a cancer that is strongly related to previous alcohol use, such as a liver cancer or head and neck cancer. This is common sense. But for breast cancer, even though many websites recommend that patients limit their alcohol intake, the data actually paints a much more nuanced picture. In one of the best studies looking at this issue,[123] women who drank less than half a serving of alcohol per day had a lower risk of cancer recurrence, as well as a lower risk of dying from breast cancer, than women who drank more. Sounds great. The downside was that the women who drank more than half a serving a day had a lower chance of dying from causes like cardiovascular disease. So, in the end, it was a wash: alcohol consumption didn't affect survival overall. It was recommended that women weigh these two potential options and come to their own decision: cut out alcohol to minimize the risk of death from breast cancer, or drink some alcohol to minimize the risk of death from cardiovascular disease.[124]

Even if some lifestyle changes don't reduce the risk of cancer recurring, they can still provide other health benefits that shouldn't be ignored. The end of cancer treatment represents an opportunity to make changes. Often this new era after treatment can include a change in lifestyle and another look at how to maximize health. It makes sense to talk to your doctors about interventions to optimize your overall health so you can minimize the risk of other important illnesses besides cancer.

Wrap-up and Mini-checklist

Survivorship is an important part of cancer care. Follow-up care has evolved from focusing only on detecting recurrences and dealing with side effects to a more holistic approach that includes prevention and early detection of new cancers, along with provision of psychological, emotional, and social supports when needed. An SCP can be an important tool to help organize your post-treatment care. The transition from treatment to follow-up also represents an opportunity to make positive life changes, such as quitting smoking, to maximize your overall health.*

Here are the main questions for your health care team:

- *Can you help me to develop a survivorship care plan?*

- *Who will be responsible for my ongoing follow-up, according to the plan I have created with my team?*

- *How often will visits and tests be necessary, and who will arrange them?*

- *Does my follow-up plan fit with current guidelines for surveillance of my type of cancer?*

- *What issues or symptoms should I bring to the attention of my health care team?*

- *Where can I turn if I experience emotional distress or depressive symptoms, or if I need spiritual care?*

- *Can you help me to quit smoking?*

- *Are there any lifestyle changes I can make to reduce the risk of this cancer coming back?*

- *What can I do to optimize my overall health?*

---

* For more resources relating to survivorship, see the American Cancer Society's "Life After Treatment" booklet, linked at http://www.qualitycancertreatment. com/a09.

Resources

Survivorship Care Plans

There are several websites that specifically offer free SCPs. Two of these include the LIVESTRONG Foundation (http://www.live strongcareplan.org) and Journey Forward (http://www.journey forward.org). Both websites use a brief questionnaire to gather information from a patient or health care provider, then produce an SCP that can be reviewed with the health care team and used for future reference.*

SCPs contain a treatment summary and a plan for ongoing follow-up. The treatment summary contains information that you should now be able to assemble yourself, after working through the previous chapters. It includes the following:

- Contact information of the doctors who treated your cancer

- The diagnosis

- The stage

- Any surgeries done, including the date and procedure

- Any chemotherapy received, including the drugs and dates

- Any radiation received, including the dose and number of fractions, location targeted in the body, and the dates

- Side effects of treatment, particularly those that haven't resolved at the end of treatment

- For some cancers, any genetic or hereditary risk factors (such as whether people in your family have had cancer) or any genetic tests

---

* For more SCP websites, see http://www.qualitycancertreatment.com/a09.

The second section of the SCP is the plan for ongoing follow-up. This includes:

- Contact information for your oncology team

- The need for any additional (adjuvant) treatment for your cancer, including the name of the treatment, duration, and expected side effects

- The schedule of follow-up visits, including who will provide follow-up and where

- Tests that are needed (CT scans, mammograms, blood tests), their frequency, and who will order them

- Any screening that is needed to detect new cancers (if it differs from the recommendation for the general population) or any other testing or examinations needed

- Possible symptoms to be aware of that could signal a return of the cancer and possible important long-term side effects of treatment

- A list of some of the other important issues that can arise (emotional, financial), with a list of resources for help and statements about the importance of other healthy lifestyle factors

CHAPTER 14

When There Is No Cure

Despite all of the advances in cancer treatment, and despite the fact that more patients are surviving their cancers than ever before, cancer still claims the lives of millions of people worldwide each year.[125] For some patients, there are unfortunately no curative treatment options for their cancer.

Incurable cancers can vary in their behavior. Some, like metastatic thyroid cancer, can be very slow growing, changing very little from year to year. Others can be very aggressive, progressing quickly in a number of months. Regardless of where a cancer falls on this spectrum, there are often several important steps that can be taken to make life better or longer, by slowing the growth of cancer, improving symptoms, and making sure that proper supports are in place.

In this chapter, I will help you navigate through some of these important steps.

Confirm the Reason for Incurability

There can be several reasons why a cancer is incurable. Most often, it is because the cancer has metastasized to other areas of the body, but it can also be because a cancer is too large to treat or remove, it doesn't respond to treatment, or the patient is too unfit for treatment.

We learned in chapter 4 that doctors usually use scans to determine whether a cancer has spread elsewhere in the body. We also learned that spots on a scan—lesions—are not always cancer. And occasionally, lesions that appear to be metastatic cancer are proven not to be cancer after all. This difference can have big implications: if a lesion that is presumed to be a metastasis is proven not to be cancer, then the patient actually has lower-stage disease (stage I, II, or III) and a curative-intent treatment might be possible.

The ultimate test to confirm the presence of metastatic cancer is usually a biopsy of a lesion that appears to be a metastasis.

Do we always need a biopsy to determine with certainty that a cancer has spread? It depends. There are situations in which the scans are quite clear and a biopsy might not be needed. If a patient with a known lung cancer develops several spots on his scans (for example, in the bones, lung, and/or brain) that are new and highly suspicious, many doctors would not suggest a biopsy, as the probability of an alternative diagnosis is very low. But when there is any uncertainty, doctors should consider getting definitive biopsy confirmation that the spots on the scans are indeed cancer.

Here are some questions to ask your doctors about your diagnosis if you are faced with an incurable cancer:

- *What is it about my cancer that makes it incurable?*

- *Do we need a biopsy to confirm that the findings on the scans truly represent metastases?*

- *Even if the cancer has spread to a few spots (like to the bone or liver), are there treatments that we can use to kill those metastatic spots?*

  - In some very select cases, guidelines suggest that aggressive treatment of the metastases should be considered when there are only a few spots of cancer, and this is an area of ongoing research.[126]

Consider a Clinical Trial

In chapter 7, we discussed the importance of knowing the goals of treatment, along with the risks and benefits of treatment in your specific situation. When a cancer is incurable, treatments may still be able to prolong life, but it's worth repeating here that in a palliative situation, both doctors and patients are less willing to compromise quality of life to initiate treatment.

When a cancer is incurable, it's especially worth considering entering a clinical trial. The main reason to join a clinical trial is that it may improve treatment options for future patients. But as we discussed when reviewing clinical trials in chapter 12, a blockbuster treatment occasionally comes along, and patients who try the treatment in a trial while it is still experimental reap the benefits (although there are no guarantees). Ask your doctors if there are any trials available to you, and if you haven't read chapter 12, read it now to learn more about types of trials and how to find them.

Treatment Choices: Strike a Balance

For many types of cancer, even if the cancer itself is incurable, there are treatments available that have been proven to extend life. The mainstay of treatment for metastatic cancers is usually systemic therapy. The use of surgery or high doses of radiation for patients in this setting is uncommon (although useful in some very specific situations).[127] More commonly, radiation is used for relieving symptoms, such as pain or cough, and is not expected to extend life, just to improve quality of life.* But systemic therapy is the major approach to treating cancers when the intent is palliative.

---

* If palliative radiation is recommended for your situation, refer to chapter 10 to read more about it. In a palliative setting, shorter courses of radiation are often warranted. As little as one treatment can be sufficient for improving pain.

When patients receive systemic therapy for palliative treatment, there is usually a pecking order of drugs that are used. The most effective and best-proven drugs are usually called "first-line" treatments. First-line treatments may be quite effective initially, but after a time, the cancer becomes resistant to that treatment, and doctors will consider moving on to "second-line" treatment. When second-line treatment fails, there can be a "third-line" treatment and, occasionally, additional options beyond that, depending on the cancer. But as doctors move down the list, the chances of a response tend to diminish. A third-line treatment is rarely as effective as a first-line treatment, not only because the drugs may not be as good, but also because the cancer will have become more resistant due to the previous treatments. This decrease in effectiveness changes the risk-benefit ratio, because even though the chances of benefit are decreasing with each subsequent line of treatment, the risk of side effects doesn't diminish and may even increase if a patient is becoming frailer. The balance between risk and benefit is more likely to be affected in a negative way.

In 2012, the American Society of Clinical Oncology launched a "Choosing Wisely" campaign to help doctors make good decisions about when to use systemic therapy in a palliative setting. The first recommendation on the list* was that doctors avoid using cancer-directed therapy (including systemic therapies) in patients with poor performance status (which we discussed in chapter 3) when there has been no benefit from prior treatments, when patients are ineligible for a clinical trial, and without strong evidence that additional treatment would help. The Choosing Wisely campaign goes on to explain this recommendation to patients:

> If you have had three different treatments and your cancer has grown
> or spread, more treatment usually will not help you feel better or

---

* Available at http://www.choosingwisely.org/societies/american-society-of-clinical
  -oncology/.

increase your chance of living longer. Instead, more treatment could cause serious side effects that shorten your life and reduce the quality of the time you have left. Still, almost half of people with advanced cancer keep getting chemotherapy—even when it has almost no chance of helping them. They end up suffering when they should not have to.[128]

Despite this advice, the literature is clear that doctors are too aggressive when it comes to treating patients when there is no chance of cure. In 2016, Ronald Chen from the University of North Carolina looked to see whether aggressive treatments were still being delivered to patients at the end of life. He and his colleagues examined records from 28,731 US patients under the age of 65 who had died of a metastatic cancer in the years between 2007 and 2014, including patients with lung, breast, colorectal, pancreatic, and prostate cancers. He found that approximately 75 percent of patients were receiving some type of aggressive intervention in the last 30 days of life, such as chemotherapy, radiotherapy, an invasive procedure, or hospital admission. Rates of admission to intensive care units, which usually reflect very aggressive care, were between 16 and 20 percent. Dr. Chen compared the rates of aggressive care before and after the Choosing Wisely campaign began, and they hadn't yet changed. They concluded: "There is substantial overuse of aggressive end-of-life care."[129]

I don't want to discount the value of treatment: for some patients, particularly those who are fit, with a good performance status, treatment can add months or even years of life, without substantially undermining quality of life. But for other patients, when previous treatments haven't worked, or if their performance status is not good, then further treatments may be more likely to cause harm. Try to strike a balance that is ideal for you.

Patients have different preferences in terms of trade-offs between risks and benefits. At one end of the spectrum, some patients are willing to take major risks, or undertake very difficult treatments, in an effort to extend life. At the other end are those who want to preserve quality of life at all costs, even if it means a shorter life overall. And there are patients at various points in between. The key is to determine where your own preferences lie on this spectrum. Discuss these wishes with people who are close to you, and communicate your preferences to your doctor.

In chapter 7, we discussed weighing the risks and benefits of treatment and the importance of knowing the goals of treatment. Some of the questions in this situation are the same, but some are different. Here are some questions to discuss with your doctors:

- *What are the goals of treatment?*

- *How much additional benefit do you expect from this treatment, in light of previous treatments?*

- *How much will this treatment affect my quality of life and in what ways?*

- *How quickly will we know if treatment is working, so I can decide whether to stop or continue?*

- *What would happen if I have no anticancer treatment?*

- *What can I expect in the future?*

- *What would lead you to recommend that we stop anticancer treatments?*

Below, we will talk about living wills, with tools to help you discuss your preferences and make decisions about the care you wish to receive.

Palliative Care: Improving and Extending Life

Palliative care is defined as specialized medical care that is aimed at relieving symptoms, including pain and stress, from any serious illness, not just cancer. The goal of palliative care is to improve quality of life—not only for the patient, but also for the patient's family.[130] In some centers, the palliative care team is referred to as the "pain and symptom management team."

Palliative care has generally been considered to mean "end-of-life care," but that is not always the case. Palliative care can be provided long before the end of life and, in some cases, even when the cancer treatment itself is not palliative. For some of my patients who have severe nausea during curative-intent treatment, I ask the palliative care team to help me manage those symptoms, as they are the experts in symptom management. And "palliative care" does not mean "giving up": even for patients with incurable cancers, palliative care can be provided along with standard anticancer treatment (like chemotherapy), rather than waiting for the end of life.*

Waiting until the very end of life to involve palliative care is generally not a good idea. Emerging data suggests that the sooner the palliative care team is involved, the better.[131] Several randomized studies have examined this issue, assigning patients with incurable cancers to one of two options: see the palliative care team immediately, or wait until their oncologists feel that their symptoms require help from the palliative care team. The results are striking. Patients who are referred immediately have a better understanding of their prognosis, a significant reduction in the intensity of their cancer

---

* When palliative care is given near the end of life, the term "hospice care" is often used in the United States. Hospice care refers to palliative care specifically within the last six months of life. The term "hospice" also refers to a specific facility where hospice care can be given, although it can also be given at home or in a hospital.

symptoms, better quality of life, and less depression. They are also less likely to receive chemotherapy near the end of life. Chemotherapy near the end of life (within the last two weeks) is generally not a desirable thing and is used as a marker of quality of care, with lower rates being better. And palliative care referrals don't lead to a shorter period of survival. In fact, the opposite appears to be true: in two randomized trials, early referral to palliative care led to longer survival compared with patients who were referred later.[132]

Palliative care can take many forms, including telephone discussions with nurses, in-person visits with doctors, and even smartphone apps. Interestingly, a recent randomized study showed that patients with advanced lung cancer who were given access to a palliative care app that tracked symptoms and reported them to their oncologists had better survival than those who did not have the app.[133]

There is no single factor in palliative care that leads to better outcomes, but there are three main mechanisms by which it is believed that the palliative care team helps: (1) by managing and improving the patient's symptoms; (2) by addressing the patient's emotions and helping the patient with coping; and (3) by enhancing communication between the patient and the oncologist.[134]

Consider asking your doctor for a referral to the palliative care team. If there are symptoms that your doctors are having difficulty controlling, such as pain, nausea, or vomiting, see the section on side effects and symptom management in chapter 11. For more information about palliative care, including an excellent list of resources, see https://getpalliativecare.org/.

Mood and Emotions

Sadness and grief are normal reactions to a diagnosis of incurable cancer. Fortunately, many cancer centers and hospitals have developed programs to help patients cope emotionally with a difficult diagnosis, and these can help to improve quality of life. Mood is important even beyond quality of life: it can affect interactions with friends and family, and it can even affect survival in ways we are only beginning to understand. A depressed mood has been associated with shorter survival in patients with incurable lung cancer.[135] In chapter 13, we discussed the importance of mood and the symptoms of depression.

Many physician visits focus on your physical health, and mental health can be an afterthought. If your mood is low, or you need help coping with any aspect of your care, bring it up with your physician or nurse. Many different interventions are available, including both medical treatments and psychological treatments. Here are some questions to ask:

- *I'd like to talk to someone about my mood. Are there counselors, social workers, spiritual care advisers, psychologists, or psychiatrists available?*

- *Are there medical treatments that can help me with my mood?*

- *Do you offer supports for my family members?*

- *Are there patient support groups I can access to talk to people who are in a similar situation?*

Your Wishes and Directives

You can specify your wishes using *advance directives*—legal documents that specify your wishes for medical care and financial issues, which often include the types of medical interventions that you want. Advance directives take two major forms: (1) a *living will*, in which you write down your preferences; and (2) a *health care proxy* or *medical power of attorney*, by which you pick someone to make decisions for you in case you are not able to do so in the future.*

A living will outlines the types of medical care that you want, or don't want, as part of your treatment. Patients can decide if they would want cardiopulmonary resuscitation, life support (such as a breathing tube placed into the lungs and attached to a machine), or a tube for feeding into the stomach.

A health care proxy or medical power of attorney directive specifies somebody to make medical decisions in case you cannot make them for yourself. Ideally, this is a person you trust, who knows your wishes, and will be available to make decisions and advocate on your behalf. This person's power kicks in only under circumstances when you can't make a decision. As long as you can make decisions for yourself, you will continue to do so.

If it happens that a patient is unable to make health care decisions but no surrogate decision maker has been specified in advance, doctors are often legally obligated to use a standard list to determine who makes decisions. First on the list is a legal guardian (if there is one), followed by the patient's spouse, then the patient's adult children, then either parent of the patient, and the list continues on from there. A problem can arise if there are multiple people at the same level who disagree. For example, for a widow with two grown children, both children would have equal say in the decision making, and if they can't agree, it can create a difficult situation. But if one person had been designated as the health care proxy, that person would go to the top of the decision-making list.

---

* The names of these two documents and their exact legal requirements vary across different states and in different countries. Ask your health care team to help you find the appropriate documents for where you live. Oncology teams often include social workers who are adept at navigating these forms.

Initially, it can seem overwhelming to have to make decisions about health care scenarios that might (or might not) arise down the road. A good place to start is with a living will document titled "Five Wishes" (described in detail at the end of this chapter). Dealing with these issues at the start of your treatment journey has the benefit of ensuring that your wishes are in place in case of unexpected events. As well, this allows you to focus on your treatment and avoids having to address these issues in a time of crisis.

Wrap-up and Mini-checklist

In this chapter, we've learned that for patients with incurable cancers, several important steps can be taken to help maximize quality and quantity of life. In a palliative setting, it is often important to confirm that the diagnosis is indeed correct, and that may require an additional biopsy. Although treatments such as chemotherapy may extend life, careful consideration of the risks and benefits of treatment is needed. After first-line treatment, the subsequent treatments are often less effective. Getting a palliative care team involved early can improve several outcomes and may even help patients live longer.

The needs of patients with advanced cancer are diverse, and not all can be covered in a single chapter. For many of the other important concerns that arise, such as financial issues, creating a legal will, and discussions with family and children, an excellent resource is the American Society of Clinical Oncology's "Advanced Cancer" web page.[*]

---

[*] See http://www.cancer.net/navigating-cancer-care/advanced-cancer.

Here is a review of some of the important questions to ask your doctor and health care team when the goal of treatment is palliative:

- *What is it about my cancer that makes it incurable?*

- *Do we need a biopsy to confirm that the spots considered to be metastases are actually cancer?*

- *Is there a clinical trial available for me?*

- *What are the goals of treatment, and how much benefit do you expect?*

- *How much will this treatment affect my quality of life?*

- *How quickly will we know if treatment is working, so I can decide whether to stop or continue?*

- *What would happen if I have no treatment?*

- *At what point do we stop anticancer treatments?*

- *Can we get a palliative care team involved in my care?*

- *What supports are available if my mood is low or if I'm depressed?*

- *Can you help me to complete my advance directives?*

Resources

Living Wills

The Five Wishes living will (available at http://www.agingwith dignity.org) helps you consider five aspects of your medical care:

1. The person you want to make care decisions for you when you can't

2. The kind of medical treatment you want or don't want

3. How comfortable you want to be

4. How you want people to treat you

5. What you want your loved ones to know

In most US states, filling out the Five Wishes document meets the legal requirement for an advance directive. In the other states, it can be attached to a legal advance directive form, which your doctor can direct you to (and which is also available on the Aging with Dignity website).

Even if the Five Wishes form is not a legal document in your state or country, you can use it as a place to start. You can bring a completed copy to your health care team to begin the discussion about creating an advance directive.

CHAPTER 15

Cancer Myths and Truths

Part of good decision making is being able to distinguish fact from fiction. Many patients report that they are inundated with information, not only from their health care team, but also from well-meaning friends and family, the Internet, and sometimes alternative health providers. The information patients receive from a variety of sources can spark both hope and fear; it can be confusing, contradictory, and overwhelming.

In this book, I've tried to give you the best advice available for taking charge of your cancer treatment within the Western medical model, or *allopathic medicine*. Our practice is based on evidence from thousands of clinical, laboratory, and public health studies involving hundreds of thousands of patients with more than 100 different cancers.

What we know about cancer and its treatment is always changing as new evidence emerges from new studies. We've learned so much, and we have so much more to learn. This lack of absolute certainty about cancer treatment can be frustrating to a patient facing a battle for his or her life. It can be tempting to believe there's another, surer way to beat cancer. Many myths about "natural" or nonallopathic cures are floating around, often with a suggestion that medical doctors are suppressing this information.

Some of these myths are basically harmless, but sometimes they can be dangerous. I still remember with sorrow a patient of mine,

Sharon, who was diagnosed with a very treatable throat cancer. Her chances of cure using a combination of radiation and chemotherapy were about 85 percent. She was persuaded by an alternative health provider that radiation and chemotherapy could not cure cancer, but that a particular series of alternative treatments could. Six months later, Sharon was in the emergency room: the tumor in her throat was much larger, and it had begun to bleed, filling her lungs with blood. Sharon was saved by our surgeons from that emergency, and, relieved, she was eager to start the chemotherapy and radiation treatment. But her cancer had spread to other parts of her body by then, and the chance for a curative treatment had been missed. Ultimately, the cancer was incurable and it took her life.

In this chapter, I'll examine some of the more common misconceptions and myths about allopathic cancer care. At the end of the chapter, I'll give you some tips to help you decide if something is true or false. You will notice that this chapter relies heavily on the important components of evidence-based medicine: clinical studies and randomized trials. If you haven't read chapter 5 yet, it would serve as a helpful introduction to the material below.

Myth or Truth? Cancer Treatments Don't Extend Life

Several alternative health care providers and websites make claims that chemotherapy and radiation are ineffective. Some go even a step further: in 2015, a natural health website called Natural News ran an article titled "Chemotherapy Kills Cancer Patients Faster than No Treatment at All."

By this point in the book, you probably know that this statement is not true. Here is just a sampling of the hundreds (or thousands) of randomized studies that have shown benefits:

- *Prostate cancer:* For men with metastatic prostate cancer, doctors tested a drug called docetaxel in addition to the hormone therapy usually used in this situation. The men who got the chemotherapy lived an extra 14 months.[136]

- *Lung cancer:* After surgery for lung cancer, adding chemotherapy improves the odds of being alive at five years by 5 percent. A modest benefit, but one that many patients would go for.[137]

- *Breast cancer:* In women with breast cancer that has been removed by surgery, adding in even the oldest type of chemotherapy after surgery increases the chances of being alive 10 years later by 5 percent. Newer chemotherapies increase the survival rate further.[138]

We now have targeted therapies and immunotherapies, as we discussed in chapter 11. The May 2001 cover of *Time* magazine featured a revolutionary targeted drug called Gleevec (imatinib). Gleevec was designed specifically for *chronic myeloid leukemia* (CML), a type of blood cancer. In CML, one important type of mutation causes the normal blood cells to keep on dividing continuously, analogous to a switch being left in the "on" position. Gleevec was engineered specifically to block that switch. When Gleevec was tried in a phase I (safety) trial, 53 out of the 54 patients who got an adequate dose had a complete response—that is, full remission of the cancer. Later randomized trials confirmed this benefit.[139]

Immunotherapy is a relatively new treatment that has already had a major impact. For patients with melanoma that has spread to other parts of the body, the immunotherapy drug nivolumab has been shown to increase the one-year survival to 73 percent, from 42 percent with older chemotherapy.[140] Immunotherapy has already revolutionized the treatment of some cancers.

Verdict: Myth, and a dangerous one. Suggesting that patients forgo treatments that are proven to help can lead to substantial harm.

Myth or Truth? Dietary Changes Can Fight Cancer

A few years ago, I was caring for a man who was near the end of his life because of metastatic lung cancer. He had tried all sorts of treatment, including radiation and chemotherapy, but ultimately, the cancer stopped responding, and we knew he had a short time to live. We spent a long time discussing his goals for end-of-life care. At the end of the discussion, he still had one last question. Given the nature of the conversation, I was expecting him to bring up a very profound question that we hadn't addressed. Instead, he asked me: "Doc, can I have a piece of chocolate cake?"

Unbeknownst to me, for the past year, he had given up sugar. He'd been told that eating sugar would feed his cancer, and he'd gone to great lengths to avoid it. Now he wanted to have some cake before he died.

Questions like this are common. Various types of dietary changes have been touted as a way to cure or slow cancer: cut out sugar, as my patient was told, but also cut out dairy or gluten, eat organic, eat vegan, or drink lots of vegetable juices. Can you eat, or diet, your way to a cure?

Most of these dietary interventions have not been formally tested in studies, but a few have been, and the results are not very positive. The dietary intervention that has the best supporting data is a low-fat diet, either for prostate cancer or breast cancer, and the effects of that intervention are very modest at best.

In prostate cancer, a low-fat diet was tested in a randomized trial of men who were undergoing active surveillance (which means

221

observation of a low-risk cancer, without treatment). The diet was part of an intensive lifestyle program including a vegan ultra-low-fat diet, vitamin supplements, exercise, and stress management (including yoga, meditation, and imagery). Compared with a control group, the effects were modest, with only a slight difference in PSA levels between the two groups.[141] This would be considered very weak evidence of a benefit: the study intervention included multiple factors, not just diet, and the "benefit" was only a small change in a blood test.

Another randomized study examined a low-fat diet in women with breast cancer and found a small difference in relapse rates: 9.8 percent of the women on the low-fat diet had a return of the cancer, compared with 12.4 percent of women on their usual diets.[142] But not all studies have shown an anticancer effect from a low-fat diet, whether for breast cancer or other cancers, so the jury is still out.[143]

For the other dietary interventions, such as restricting sugar, there just isn't good evidence that these affect relapse rates of cancer.[144] Although some observational studies suggest that dietary patterns may be associated with recurrence rates,[145] this association does not establish cause and effect. We need randomized trials to prove that dietary interventions work before we can recommend them.

There can be some downsides to restrictive diets: they can lead to unnecessary weight loss (which can be dangerous if patients are also losing weight due to treatment or their cancer), and patients may feel increased stress or guilt when trying to follow a difficult diet.

Verdict: For most dietary interventions, myth. For low-fat diets in prostate cancer and breast cancer patients, there may be a very modest benefit, but the evidence is weak. It is important, for other health reasons, to stick to a healthy diet. But clear proof that dietary interventions can keep cancer away—or cure it—is lacking. My answer to that patient? Eat the cake!

Myth or Truth? Alternative Treatments Can Cure Cancer

A web search for alternative treatments for cancer leads to several options, with claims that sound promising. These include vitamin C or other antioxidants, homeopathy, ozone therapy, and making your body less acidic.

The truth is that none of these approaches has been shown to have any effect on cancer in humans. Many alternative approaches have not been formally studied, but some have. Let's look at some of these ideas.

Vitamin C is an *antioxidant,* a type of chemical found in oranges and other fruits and vegetables.[146] Antioxidants are compounds that prevent oxygen-related chemicals from damaging our cells.[147] They have been touted as being useful to prevent or treat cancer, but this has not been borne out in human studies—in fact, they have sometimes been shown to be harmful. Although vitamin C has shown some promise in animal and laboratory studies, randomized trials of vitamin C, with or without other antioxidants, in human cancer patients haven't shown anticancer effects.[148] Antioxidants may actually accelerate cancer progression, which was demonstrated in a randomized trial that used the antioxidant beta-carotene to prevent lung cancer. The patients who received the beta-carotene actually developed more cancers than those who received a placebo.[149]

Homeopathy is generally based on the practice of taking a compound that in a healthy person would cause the same symptoms as the disease being treated, diluting it an extreme number of times so there is essentially nothing left, and then administering the diluted liquid to a patient. A recent review by the Australian National Health and Medical Research Council found that there is no evidence to suggest that homeopathy is better than placebo for any human health condition, including cancer.[150]

Ozone therapy is touted online as a way of improving delivery of oxygen to tumors, but there have been very few studies in cancer patients, and none have been randomized.[151] There is no proof that ozone has any impact on cancer in humans.

The principle of **alkalinization** holds that cancer cells can't grow in an alkaline environment. The term "alkaline" refers to a substance (in this case, the blood) that has a pH of greater than 7. The pH scale specifies whether a chemical is an acid (with a pH less than 7) or a base (pH greater than 7). Human blood usually has a pH of around 7.4. The theory is that by ingesting alkaline substances, the pH goes up and the cancer cannot grow. There are a few problems with this theory, including the fact that the body tries to regulate pH very tightly and will always work to bring pH back to a normal value, so pH changes are temporary at best. More importantly, no studies have indicated that alkalinization can fight cancer in humans.

Despite this lack of proven benefit for these interventions, some alternative practitioners continue to support their use. This highlights one of the fundamental differences between alternative medical practitioners and medical doctors: the need for evidence. As an oncologist, even if I believe a new compound is effective against cancer, I would not prescribe it (and nor would my colleagues) without evidence suggesting a benefit. As a profession, medical doctors strive to design trials to prove that new treatments work, so we can benefit patients now and in the future. Alternative medical practitioners don't abide by that philosophy.

Alternative treatments are not without risk. Like any compound you put into your body, there may be unintended side effects. A national study done in Norway compared survival in patients who used alternative medicines with those who did not, and it suggested that use of alternatives was associated with *worse* survival, particularly in patients with the best performance status (that is, those who were highest-functioning).[152] A separate study of patients in Korea who had incurable cancers showed that the use of alternative medicines didn't appear to impact survival either way, but it was associated with worse cognitive functioning and more fatigue. Several different types of alternative medicines appeared to worsen quality of life in some way, including vitamins, mushrooms, and other dietary interventions.[153]

There are other downsides, including the increased cost of alternative medicines and the fact that providing false hope can lead to patients making poor decisions. The worst example of this is when patients forgo a potentially curative treatment to try something alternative and then miss the window of opportunity for cure. This is what happened to Sharon, described above, and also to Steve Jobs, the founder of Apple. Jobs's cancer journey was well publicized, with media reports indicating that he refused a potentially curative treatment to pursue dietary and other alternative methods, a decision he came to regret, according to his biographer. By the time he changed his mind, the cancer had spread.*

Verdict: Myth.**

---

* The full account of Jobs's story is linked at http://www.qualitycancertreatment .com/a10.

** There is a directory with information about specific alternative health products on the NCI website at https://www.cancer.gov/about-cancer/treatment/cam /patient. To read the perspective of a former naturopath on the value of naturopathic medicine in cancer care, go to http://www.qualitycancertreatment.com /blog/naturopathictreatment.

Myth or Truth? Doctors Are Hiding a Cure

The premise with this statement is that since doctors make a living from treating cancer, if there was a cure, we'd all be hitting the unemployment lines. So we just clam up and keep the cure to ourselves.

There's one obvious problem with this logic: doctors and their family members die of cancer too. I have lost colleagues to cancer, and some of my colleagues have lost spouses and children. If there were a cure that we were not sharing with the public, certainly we would use it for ourselves and our loved ones.

Does it seem logical that an oncologist would let his child die, or die himself, just to keep a secret cure hidden? No sane person would do that. It just doesn't make sense.

Verdict: Myth.

Myth or Truth: Pharmaceutical Companies Are Hiding the Cure

In this version, the doctors are blameless, but the magic bullet is hidden by a greedy pharmaceutical company that wants to keep the real cure hidden so it can continue to sell drugs that don't work as well.

Let's consider the economics of this. We'll imagine that a pharmaceutical company has a magic bullet, a single pill that will cure all cancers. Is it better to sell the single pill or to sell less-effective treatments that patients have to keep taking for years?

Governments and insurers pay a lot of money for medical treatments. In many countries, the decision about how much to pay for a drug (or whether to pay for it at all) depends on its benefit compared to the cost. A drug that increases someone's life span by 10 years is worth much more than a drug that gets only an extra month.

To calculate if a drug is worth paying for, health economists use a value called the *quality-adjusted life year*, or QALY. If a drug adds one year of high-quality time to your life (in other words, during that extra year, you are not sick with side effects or disabled), it adds one QALY. This allows payers to decide which medical treatments are worth funding. If one treatment costs $100,000 per QALY and another costs $500,000 per QALY, it makes sense to prioritize the cheaper one over the more expensive one.

Some countries draw a line in the sand dictating the maximum they will pay per extra QALY. A cost of $100,000 per QALY is a reasonable line. If a new drug comes along that costs $500,000 per QALY, it would not be funded with that cutoff. Some countries have higher or lower cutoffs or no cutoff at all.

If we were willing to pay $100,000 per QALY, we can calculate the value of that magic bullet hidden by a drug company. If you give the magic bullet to a 30-year-old patient who is about to pass away from a terminal cancer, she would be cured and might be expected to live to age 80. As long as she has good quality of life, you've given her 50 extra QALYs, and the drug company could reasonably charge $5 million ($100,000 per QALY x 50 QALYs). If, instead, the drug company offered a series of drugs that kept the patient alive for five years, the most it could get under this system would be $500,000.

With those numbers, the economic value of a magic bullet would be staggering. Keeping a magic bullet locked away in a safe would be the worst business model of all time.

Verdict: Myth.

Myth or Truth? Pharmaceutical Companies Influence Physicians

Pharmaceutical companies and medical device companies are involved in many aspects of cancer: drug and device development, including basic science research to develop new compounds, running clinical trials, and marketing. These companies inherently have a conflict of interest: they are tasked with running unbiased studies with scientific integrity, but they also have a motive to generate revenue and profits.

Pharmaceutical companies play an integral role in developing new treatments and bringing them to patients, but because of their commercial focus, many of their actions are not in the best interests of patients. The types of unsavory behaviors are many.

First, they inflate the costs of medications. It's been well established that drug prices are much too high, and they don't reflect the true cost of drug development.[154] The cost of a new cancer medication is often more than $100,000 per year per patient. Before the year 2000, average prices for all new cancer drugs were less than $10,000 per year.[155]

Second, pharmaceutical companies can impact the results of trials. Industry-sponsored trials, whether they are examining drugs or new devices, are more likely to show results favorable to the new drug or device being tested.[156] Sometimes negative trials are suppressed.[157]

Third, they influence physician behavior, as we discussed in chapter 6.

There are several initiatives under way to try to stop these practices. Requirements are now in place that mandate that all clinical trials must be registered prior to starting,[158] so physicians can more easily spot "missing trials" that may be suppressed. New requirements as of 2016 will stipulate that the raw patient data from clinical trials must also be made public after publication of the study results, so the results can be double-checked.[159]

Additionally, researchers must now declare their own personal conflicts of interest when submitting new research or giving presentations. New laws and regulations are limiting the ability of companies to meet with doctors or to provide gifts. In the United States, the Physician Payments Sunshine Act[160] requires that manufacturers who participate in federal health care programs report payments and certain gifts to physicians and that data must be entered into a searchable database.* But there is still much work to be done.

Verdict: Truth. The risk of potential influence is very real, and the profession needs to continue to work to ensure that safeguards are in place to protect against this.

Myth or Truth? We've Made No Progress in the Fight Against Cancer

Millions of dollars are spent on cancer research every year, yet cancer is still a killer. If you read certain websites or social media posts, people might claim that we're no further ahead than we were many years ago. Has the money been for nothing?

Fortunately, we have some good data examining survival rates for cancer patients going back several decades.[161] We can boil it down to a simple question. Who would survive longer: a patient diagnosed with cancer back in 1975 or a patient diagnosed more recently?

For patients diagnosed with cancer in 1975, only 49 percent were still alive five years later. But for patients diagnosed in 2010, that number jumps up to 69 percent. Instead of more than half of patients dying before five years, it's now less than one-third. Other countries, including Canada, have achieved similar results.[162]

---

* You can look up a doctor or hospital here: https://www.cms.gov/openpayments/.

Table 6. US Data for Specific Cancers

Type of Cancer	Patients Diagnosed in 1975–77 Surviving ≥ 5 Years	Patients Diagnosed in 2005–11 Surviving ≥ 5 Years
Breast cancer	75%	91%
Prostate cancer	68%	99%
Colon cancer	50%	66%
Leukemia	34%	62%
Lung cancer	12%	18%
Pancreatic cancer	3%	8%

Table 6 shows data for a handful of cancers. We can see some enormous improvements and also some more modest ones. For some cancers, even though the numbers are better, the survival remains low. But if someone tells you that we're not making any progress against cancer, tell them it's not true.

Verdict: Myth.

How to Decipher Fact from Fiction

How do you evaluate a claim about a treatment that sounds promising? Below are some tips for trying to help you decide if a treatment is actually useful. For some real-life examples of how to determine if medical claims seem reasonable, see the "Distinguishing Myths from

Truths" video in the Patient Toolkit (http://www.qualitycancertreatment.com/toolkit).

- Consider the source. A major academic hospital is more reliable than an unknown blogger.

- Check the backstory. Scientific writers will use references, just as I have. If there are no references, that can be a red flag. If there are references, have a look and see how strong those studies are and if they look reputable.

- Check the scientific literature. Use the resources in chapter 8 to see what the science says about the particular treatments.

- Anecdotes are not reliable. People may claim to have been cured by all types of different treatments, but those claims may not be true.

- Be wary of people who are promising the world. If it sounds too good to be true, it probably is.

- If an alternative health care practitioner asks you to keep something secret or not discuss it with your oncology team, that is a big red flag.

- Ask your doctor about any alternative treatment you might be considering. Most doctors are very open to discussing new ideas and alternative treatments and will appreciate being informed.

The *Taking Charge of Cancer* Patient Checklist

This concluding section of the book contains the *Taking Charge of Cancer* Patient Checklist. You can use this resource as a guide to make sure that many of the major issues in this book have been addressed in your care. Not all of the issues in the book are covered here, so it should not be considered a replacement for reading the earlier chapters in this book. For each of the items below, refer to the previous chapters for more details.

I hope this book has been helpful to you. Writing it has been a volunteer effort, as any royalties that would come to me are being donated to cancer research. If you have further questions, talk to your doctors, check some of the patient resources covered throughout this book, or post a question on the Quality Cancer Treatment website (http://www.qualitycancertreatment.com). You can also submit comments there, to let me know if this book has impacted you in some way. I'd like to hear from you.

Sincerely,

David Palma, MD, PhD

The *Taking Charge of Cancer* Patient Checklist

☐ I understand what cancer is and how it is generally treated.

☐ I have obtained my medical records and I understand them.

☐ I know my diagnosis, including the specific type of cancer that I have.

☐ I know the stage of my cancer, including the T-, N-, and M-stage. I know why that stage has been assigned based on my investigations, and I have checked that all the proper staging tests have been done.

☐ I understand the treatment options that are generally recommended for patients with this stage of cancer, and I have confirmed these by checking guidelines.

☐ I have a good understanding of the goals of treatment (curative or palliative) and the risks and benefits of treatment.

☐ I have considered obtaining additional opinions. This could include MDT review, other types of review, online resources, and/or review by other doctors.

☐ I am confident that all aspects of my treatment (surgery, radiation, and/or systemic therapy) are being delivered in a high-quality manner, based on reading chapters 9–11.

☐ I have discussed the option of clinical trials with my doctor. I know that the NCCN believes that the best treatment for any patient is through a clinical trial.

☐ I have asked my health care team about any other resources that are important to me, including medical, financial, and emotional supports.

☐ I have a detailed understanding of my follow-up plans after treatment, including visits, scans, timing, and who will carry these out. I have checked these against published guidelines.

☐ If applicable, I have discussed my wishes for end-of-life care with my loved ones and designated a power of attorney.

☐ I have researched any alternative treatments with reliable evidence-based resources and discussed them with my oncology team.

Acknowledgments

This book would not have been possible without the ideas and support of my wife, Dr. Cheryl Smits. She encouraged me to write about something that I'm passionate about, to assemble a book that would be helpful for patients. My children, Kiara, Adam, and William, are a daily reminder of what is truly important in life. Their presence has inspired me to see this project through, to try to create a book that might help others be successful in their fight against cancer and therefore be able to enjoy more of the important things in life as well. I am thankful to my parents, Enzo and Andrena Palma, and to my brother, Mark, for their never-ending love and support.

I've had many inspiring mentors in medicine. Although there are too many to name them all here, I want to thank those who have had the most profound impact at critical junctures in my life: Drs. Tom Pickles, Mira Keyes, and Scott Tyldesley in Vancouver; Drs. Suresh Senan and Ben Slotman in Amsterdam; Drs. Glenn Bauman and George Rodrigues in London; and two others who have passed away, Dr. Francis Chan and Dr. Barry Sheehan. Dr. Anthony Zietman, who wrote the foreword to this book, is a giant in the field of oncology and a pioneer in cancer care. I am deeply grateful for his contribution. I also thank Dr. Alex Louie, a close friend and a stellar cancer researcher. He provided crucial insight for this book, as well as for many of my research projects and other life endeavors. To the many more physicians, researchers, and health care team members who have helped to teach and guide me over the years, please know that I am thankful to all of you.

I thank all the readers who helped me shape my message by reading parts of this book, including Robert Jez, Andrew Warner, Richard McClelland, Alison Brown, Dr. Glenn Bauman, Dr. Alison Allan, Dr. Anthony Nichols, Dr. Muriel Brackstone, Dr. Shiraz Malik, Dr. Stewart Gaede, Dr. Keith Kwan, Dr. Simon Lo, Dr. Mark Landis, and, of course, my wife. I also thank my editorial team at New Harbinger, including Jess O'Brien, Clancy Drake, and Cindy Nixon, and my outstanding agent, Jill Marsal, who collectively, and very professionally, helped sculpt my writing into the book you hold in your hands.

Notes

1   The impact of hospital volume, surgeon volume, and other surgical practices on outcomes is discussed and referenced in chapter 9.

2   The impact of radiation quality on outcomes is discussed and referenced in chapter 10.

3   We will discuss appropriate staging—and studies showing that in many cases it's not being done—in chapter 4; these studies are discussed and referenced there.

4   Hewitt, M., and J. Simone, eds. 1999. *Ensuring Quality Cancer Care.* National Academies Press, pp. 2, 4. http://www.nap.edu/catalog/6467 /ensuring-quality-cancer-care.

5   Spinks, T., et al. 2012. "Ensuring Quality Cancer Care: A Follow-Up Review of the Institute of Medicine's Ten Recommendations for Improving the Quality of Cancer Care in America." *Cancer* 118(10): 2571–82.

6   DeVita, V. T., Jr., and E. DeVita-Raeburn. 2015. *The Death of Cancer: After Fifty Years on the Front Lines of Medicine, a Pioneering Oncologist Reveals Why the War on Cancer Is Winnable—and How We Can Get There.* New York: Sarah Crighton Books, pp. 20, 241. This is one of the best cancer books I've read; in fact, I read it cover to cover in 24 hours.

7   For an excellent reference covering the material in this chapter, see DeVita, V. T., Jr., T. S. Lawrence, and S. A. Rosenberg, eds. 2011. *DeVita, Hellman, and Rosenberg's Cancer: Principles & Practice of Oncology.* 9th ed. Philadelphia: Lippincott Williams & Wilkins. For more on the Hallmarks of Cancer, see Hanahan, D., and R. A. Weinberg. 2011. "Hallmarks of Cancer: The Next Generation." *Cell* 144: 646–74. For the function of normal cells, see Lodish, H., et al. 2012. *Molecular Cell Biology.* 7th ed. New York: W. H. Freeman and Company.

8   Marusyk, A., and K. Polyak. 2010. "Tumor Heterogeneity: Causes and Consequences." *Biochimica et Biophysica Acta* 1805: 105–17.

9   Gabrijel, S., et al. 2008. "Receiving the Diagnosis of Lung Cancer: Patient Recall of Information and Satisfaction with Physician Communication." *Journal of Clinical Oncology* 26: 297–302.

10 Pitkethly, M., S. MacGillivray, and R. Ryan. 2008. "Recordings or Summaries of Consultations for People with Cancer." *Cochrane Database of Systematic Reviews*. http://dx.doi.org/10.1002/14651858.CD001539.pub2.

11 Groopman, J. 2007. *How Doctors Think*. New York: Houghton Mifflin, p. 174. Many of the themes that are discussed in chapters 5 and 6 are discussed in more detail in this book.

12 For evidence supporting the benefits of accessing medical records and the rates at which patients access their records, see Ross, S. E., and C. T. Lin. 2003. "The Effects of Promoting Patient Access to Medical Records: A Review." *Journal of the American Medical Informatics Association* 10: 129–38; Walker, J., et al. 2011. "Inviting Patients to Read Their Doctors' Notes: Patients and Doctors Look Ahead: Patient and Physician Surveys." *Annals of Internal Medicine* 155(12): 811–19; and Ferreira, A., et al. 2007. "Why Facilitate Patient Access to Medical Records." *Studies in Health Technolology and Informatics* 127: 77–90.

13 For example, you can see the Canadian Medical Association's policy on medical records at https://www.cma.ca/Assets/assets-library/document/en/PD00–06-e.pdf.

14 See Cane, P., et al. 2016. "The LungPath Study: Variation in the Diagnostic and Staging Pathway for Patients with Lung Cancer in England." *Thorax* 71(3): 291–93. See also Faris, N., et al. 2015. "Preoperative Evaluation of Lung Cancer in a Community Health Care Setting." *Annals of Thoracic Surgery* 100: 394–400.

15 See Simos, D., et al. 2015. "Imaging for Distant Metastases in Women with Early-Stage Breast Cancer: A Population-Based Cohort Study." *Canadian Medical Association Journal* 187: E387–97; and Cooperberg, M. R., et al. 2002. "Contemporary Trends in Imaging Test Utilization for Prostate Cancer Staging: Data from the Cancer of the Prostate Strategic Urologic Research Endeavor." *Journal of Urology* 168(2): 491–95.

16 Simos, D., B. Hutton, and M. Clemons. 2015. "Are Physicians Choosing Wisely When Imaging for Distant Metastases in Women with Operable Breast Cancer?" *Journal of Oncology Practice* 11(1): 62–68.

17   Smith, G. C. S., and J. P. Pell. 2003. "Parachute Use to Prevent Death
     and Major Trauma Related to Gravitational Challenge: Systematic
     Review of Randomised Controlled Trials." *British Medical Journal*
     327(7429): 1459–61.

18   Sanson-Fisher, R. W., et al. 2007. "Limitations of the Randomized Con-
     trolled Trial in Evaluating Population-Based Health Interventions."
     American Journal of Preventative Medicine 33(2): 155–61.

19   Wallace, K., et al. 2006. "Impact of a Multi-disciplinary Patient Educa-
     tion Session on Accrual to a Difficult Clinical Trial: The Toronto Expe-
     rience with the Surgical Prostatectomy Versus Interstitial Radiation
     Intervention Trial." *Journal of Clinical Oncology* 24(25): 4158–62.

20   For example, the 2016 NCCN Guidelines allow for both as treatment
     options for low-risk prostate cancer, in addition to active surveillance or
     external radiation. You can see the guidelines at https://www.nccn.org/
     professionals/physician_gls/f_guidelines.asp.

21   Hopmans, W., et al. 2015. "Differences Between Pulmonologists, Tho-
     racic Surgeons and Radiation Oncologists in Deciding on the Treatment
     of Stage I Non-Small Cell Lung Cancer: A Binary Choice Experiment."
     Radiotherapy and Oncology 115(3): 361–66.

22   Fowler, F. J., Jr., et al. 2000. "Comparison of Recommendations by Urol-
     ogists and Radiation Oncologists for Treatment of Clinically Localized
     Prostate Cancer." *Journal of the American Medical Association* 283(24):
     3217–22.

23   For data showing how doctors tend to overestimate side effects from
     other specialties' treatments and underestimate side effects overall, see
     Kim, S. P., et al. 2014. "Specialty Bias in Treatment Recommendations
     and Quality of Life Among Radiation Oncologists and Urologists for
     Localized Prostate Cancer." *Prostate Cancer and Prostatic Diseases* 17(2):
     163–69.

24   See Sommers, B. D., et al. 2008. "Predictors of Patient Preferences and
     Treatment Choices for Localized Prostate Cancer." *Cancer* 113(8):
     2058–67; and Jang, T. L., et al. 2010. "Physician Visits Prior to Treat-
     ment for Clinically Localized Prostate Cancer." *Archives of Internal Med-
     icine* 170(5): 440–50.

25   For a commentary on this topic of physician-driven treatment choice,
     see Barry, M. J. 2010. "The Prostate Cancer Treatment Bazaar: Comment

on 'Physician Visits Prior to Treatment for Clinically Localized Prostate Cancer.'" *Archives of Internal Medicine* 170(5): 450–52.

26   In Treasure, T., R. C. Rintoul, and F. Macbeth. 2015. "SABR in Early Operable Lung Cancer: Time for Evidence." *Lancet Oncology* 16(6): 597–98.

27   Newcomer, L. N. 2012. "Changing Physician Incentives for Cancer Care to Reward Better Patient Outcomes Instead of Use of More Costly Drugs." *Health Affairs (Millwood)* 31(4): 780–85.

28   See Jacobson, M., et al. 2010. "How Medicare's Payment Cuts for Cancer Chemotherapy Drugs Changed Patterns of Treatment." *Health Affairs (Millwood)* 29(7): 1391–99; and Polite, B., R. M. Conti, and J. C. Ward. 2015. "Reform of the Buy-and-Bill System for Outpatient Chemotherapy Care Is Inevitable: Perspectives from an Economist, a Realpolitik, and an Oncologist." *American Society of Clinical Oncology Education Book,* e75–80.

29   Baker, H. 2015. "Overtreatment in Stage IV Lung Cancer in the USA." *Lancet Oncology* 16(15): e532.

30   For more on robotic surgery, see Barbash, G. I., and S. A. Glied. 2010. "New Technology and Health Care Costs: The Case of Robot-Assisted Surgery." *New England Journal of Medicine* 363(8): 701–74; and Delaney, C. P., A. J. Senagore, and L. Ponsky. 2010. "Robot-Assisted Surgery and Health Care Costs." *New England Journal of Medicine* 363(22): 2175 (author reply on 2176).

31   Halperin, E. C., P. Hutchison, and R. C. Barrier, Jr. 2004. "A Population-Based Study of the Prevalence and Influence of Gifts to Radiation Oncologists from Pharmaceutical Companies and Medical Equipment Manufacturers." *International Journal of Radiation Oncology, Biology, Physics* 59(5): 1477–83.

32   Spurling, G. K., et al. 2010. "Information from Pharmaceutical Companies and the Quality, Quantity, and Cost of Physicians' Prescribing: A Systematic Review." *PLoS Medicine* 7(10): e1000352.

33   Choudhry, N. K., R. H. Fletcher, and S. B. Soumerai. 2005. "Systematic Review: The Relationship Between Clinical Experience and Quality of Health Care." *Annals of Internal Medicine* 142(4): 260–73.

34   Ibid.

35   Slevin, M. L., et al. 1990. "Attitudes to Chemotherapy: Comparing Views of Patients with Cancer with Those of Doctors, Nurses, and General Public." *British Medical Journal* 300(6737): 1458–60.

36   Ibid.

37   McQuellon, R. P., et al. 1995. "Patient Preferences for Treatment of Metastatic Breast Cancer: A Study of Women with Early-Stage Breast Cancer." *Journal of Clinical Oncology* 13(4): 858–68.

38   Weeks, J. C., et al. 2012. "Patients' Expectations About Effects of Chemotherapy for Advanced Cancer." *New England Journal of Medicine* 367(17): 1616–25.

39   Hagerty, R. G., et al. 2005. "Communicating Prognosis in Cancer Care: A Systematic Review of the Literature." *Annals of Oncology* 16(7): 1005–53.

40   Ibid; Back, A. L., and R. M. Arnold. 2006. "Discussing Prognosis: 'How Much Do You Want to Know?' Talking to Patients Who Are Prepared for Explicit Information." *Journal of Clinical Oncology* 24(25): 4209–13; and Enzinger, A. C., et al. 2015. "Outcomes of Prognostic Disclosure: Associations with Prognostic Understanding, Distress, and Relationship with Physician Among Patients with Advanced Cancer." *Journal of Clinical Oncology* 33(32): 3809–16.

41   Weeks, J. C., et al. 1998. "Relationship Between Cancer Patients' Predictions of Prognosis and Their Treatment Preferences." *Journal of the American Medical Association* 279(21): 1709–14.

42   Enzinger et al. 2015. "Outcomes of Prognostic Disclosure."

43   Simmonds, P. C. 2000. "Palliative Chemotherapy for Advanced Colorectal Cancer: Systematic Review and Meta-Analysis." *British Medical Journal* 321(7260): 531–35.

44   Heinemann, V., et al. 2014. "FOLFIRI Plus Cetuximab Versus FOLFIRI Plus Bevacizumab as First-Line Treatment for Patients with Metastatic Colorectal Cancer (FIRE-3): A Randomised, Open-Label, Phase 3 Trial." *Lancet Oncology* 15(10): 1065–75.

45   Bismark, M. M., et al. 2012. "Legal Disputes over Duties to Disclose Treatment Risks to Patients: A Review of Negligence Claims and Complaints in Australia." *PLoS Medicine* 9(8): e1001283.

46   Xu, J., et al. 2016. "Deaths: Final Data from 2013." *National Vital Statistics Reports* 64(2). http://www.cdc.gov/nchs/data/nvsr/nvsr64/nvsr64_02 .pdf.

47   LaPar, D. J., et al. 2012. "The Society of Thoracic Surgeons General Thoracic Surgery Database: Establishing Generalizability to National Lung Cancer Resection Outcomes." *Annals of Thoracic Surgery* 94(1): 216–21.

48   Murray, B. 2012. "Informed Consent: What Must a Physician Disclose to a Patient?" *Virtual Mentor* 14(7): 563–66.

49   Pillay, B., et al. 2016. "The Impact of Multidisciplinary Team Meetings on Patient Assessment, Management and Outcomes in Oncology Settings: A Systematic Review of the Literature." *Cancer Treatment Reviews* 42: 56–72.

50   Brännström, F., et al. 2015. "Multidisciplinary Team Conferences Promote Treatment According to Guidelines in Rectal Cancer." *Acta Oncologica* 54(4): 447–53.

51   For some discussion on quantifying the possible benefits of tumor boards, see Devitt, B., J. Philip, and S. McLachlan. 2013. "Re: Tumor Boards and the Quality of Cancer Care." *Journal of the National Cancer Institute* 105(23): 1838; and Keating, N. L., et al. 2012. "Tumor Boards and the Quality of Cancer Care." *Journal of the National Cancer Institute* 105(2): 113–21.

52   Raab, S. S., et al. 2005. "Clinical Impact and Frequency of Anatomic Pathology Errors in Cancer Diagnoses." *Cancer* 104(10): 2205–13.

53   Talaga, T. 2010. "Mistaken Mastectomies Spark Probe of Hospital." *Toronto Star*, February 26.

54   Kennecke, H. F., et al. 2012. "Impact of Routine Pathology Review on Treatment for Node-Negative Breast Cancer." *Journal of Clinical Oncology* 30(18): 2227–31.

55   Lauritzen, P. M., et al. 2016. "Double Reading of Current Chest CT Examinations: Clinical Importance of Changes to Radiology Reports." *European Journal of Radiology* 85(1): 199–204.

56   O'Keeffe, M. M., T. M. Davis, and K. Siminoski. 2016. "Performance Results for a Workstation-Integrated Radiology Peer Review Quality Assurance Program." *International Journal for Quality in Health Care* 28(3): 294–98.

57   Kronz, J. D., W. H. Westra, and J. I. Epstein. 1999. "Mandatory Second
      Opinion Surgical Pathology at a Large Referral Hospital." *Cancer* 86(11):
      2426–35; and Tomaszewski, J. E., and V. A. LiVolsi. 1999. "Mandatory
      Second Opinion of Pathologic Slides." *Cancer* 86(11): 2198–200.

58   Meyer, A. N., H. Singh, and M. L. Graber. 2015. "Evaluation of Out-
      comes from a National Patient-Initiated Second-Opinion Program."
      American Journal of Medicine 128(10): 1138.e25–33; Payne, V. L., et al.
      "Patient-Initiated Second Opinions: Systematic Review of Characteris-
      tics and Impact on Diagnosis, Treatment, and Satisfaction." *Mayo Clinic
      Proceedings* 89(5): 687–96; and Ruetters, D., et al. 2015. "Is There Evi-
      dence for a Better Health Care for Cancer Patients After a Second
      Opinion? A Systematic Review." *Journal of Cancer Research and Clinical
      Oncology,* 142(7): 1521–1528.

59   Meyer, Singh, and Graber. 2015. "Evaluation of Outcomes."

60   Birkmeyer, J. D., et al. 2002. "Hospital Volume and Surgical Mortality in
      the United States." *New England Journal of Medicine* 346(15): 1128–37.

61   For specific data on hospital volume and outcome, see Brusselaers, N., F.
      Mattsson, and J. Lagergren. 2014. "Hospital and Surgeon Volume in
      Relation to Long-Term Survival After Oesophagectomy: Systematic
      Review and Meta-Analysis." *Gut* 63(9): 1393–400; Nuttall, M., et al.
      2004. "A Systematic Review and Critique of the Literature Relating
      Hospital or Surgeon Volume to Health Outcomes for 3 Urological
      Cancer Procedures." *Journal of Urolology* 172(6, pt. 1): 2145–52; Gooiker,
      G. A., et al. 2011. "Systematic Review and Meta-Analysis of the Volume–
      Outcome Relationship in Pancreatic Surgery." *British Journal of Surgery*
      98(4): 485–94; and Chowdhury, M. M., H. Dagash, and A. Pierro. 2007.
      "A Systematic Review of the Impact of Volume of Surgery and Special-
      ization on Patient Outcome." *British Journal of Surgery* 94(2): 145–61.

62   Dorrance, H. R., G. M. Docherty, and P. J. O'Dwyer. 2000. "Effect of
      Surgeon Specialty Interest on Patient Outcome After Potentially Cura-
      tive Colorectal Cancer Surgery." *Diseases of the Colon and Rectum* 43(4):
      492–98.

63   Goodney, P. P., et al. 2005. "Surgeon Specialty and Operative Mortality
      with Lung Resection." *Annals of Surgery* 241(1): 179–84; and Silvestri,
      G. A., et al. 1998. "Specialists Achieve Better Outcomes Than General-
      ists for Lung Cancer Surgery." *Chest* 114(3): 675–80.

64   Birkmeyer, J. D., et al. 2003. "Surgeon Volume and Operative Mortality in the United States." *New England Journal of Medicine* 349(22): 2117–27.

65   Vickers, A. J., et al. 2007. "The Surgical Learning Curve for Prostate Cancer Control After Radical Prostatectomy." *Journal of the National Cancer Institute* 99(15): 1171–77.

66   Vickers, A. J., et al. 2009. "The Surgical Learning Curve for Laparoscopic Radical Prostatectomy: A Retrospective Cohort Study." *Lancet Oncology* 10(5): 475–80.

67   Chowdhury, Dagash, and Pierro. 2007. "A Systematic Review."

68   Doolen, T., R. Nicolalde, and K. Funk. "Improper Checklist Use as a Factor in Aircraft Accidents and Incidents." http://flightdeck.ie.orst.edu /ElectronicChecklist/HTML/accidents.html.

69   World Alliance for Patient Safety. 2008. "WHO Surgical Safety Checklist." http://www.who.int/patientsafety/safesurgery/ss_checklist/en/.

70   Haynes, A. B., et al. 2009. "A Surgical Safety Checklist to Reduce Morbidity and Mortality in a Global Population." *New England Journal of Medicine* 360(5): 491–99.

71   Chaudhary, N., et al. 2015. "Implementation of a Surgical Safety Checklist and Postoperative Outcomes: A Prospective Randomized Controlled Study." *Journal of Gastrointestinal Surgery* 19(5): 935–42; and Bergs, J., et al. 2014. "Systematic Review and Meta-Analysis of the Effect of the World Health Organization Surgical Safety Checklist on Postoperative Complications." *British Journal of Surgery* 101(3): 150–58.

72   Urbach, D. R., et al. 2014. "Introduction of Surgical Safety Checklists in Ontario, Canada." *New England Journal of Medicine* 370(11): 1029–38.

73   De Vries, E. N., et al. 2010. "Effect of a Comprehensive Surgical Safety System on Patient Outcomes." *New England Journal of Medicine* 363(20): 1928–37; and Arriaga, A. F., et al. 2013. "Simulation-Based Trial of Surgical-Crisis Checklists." *New England Journal of Medicine* 368(3): 246–53.

74   Haynes, A. B., et al. 2011. "Changes in Safety Attitude and Relationship to Decreased Postoperative Morbidity and Mortality Following Implementation of a Checklist-Based Surgical Safety Intervention." *BMJ Quality & Safety* 20(1): 102–7.

75   Arriaga et al. 2013. "Simulation-Based Trial."

76 Kampf, G., H. Loffler, and P. Gastmeier. 2009. "Hand Hygiene for the Prevention of Nosocomial Infections." *Deutsches Ärzteblatt International* 106(40): 649–55; and Serkey, J. M., and G. S. Hall. 2001. "Handwashing Compliance: What Works?" *Cleveland Clinic Journal of Medicine* 68(4): 325–29, 333–34, 336.

77 Ibid.

78 Pignon, J.-P., et al. 2008. "Lung Adjuvant Cisplatin Evaluation: A Pooled Analysis by the LACE Collaborative Group." *Journal of Clinical Oncology* 26(21): 3552–59.

79 Baskar, R., et al. 2012. "Cancer and Radiation Therapy: Current Advances and Future Directions." *International Journal of Medical Sciences* 9(3): 193–99.

80 See Hoppe, B. S., et al. 2008. "Acute Skin Toxicity Following Stereotactic Body Radiation Therapy for Stage I Non-Small-Cell Lung Cancer: Who's at Risk?" *International Journal of Radiation Oncology, Biology, Physics* 72(5): 1283–86; and Furman, M. J., et al. 2013. "Gastric Perforation Following Stereotactic Body Radiation Therapy of Hepatic Metastasis from Colon Cancer." *Practical Radiation Oncology* 3(1): 10–11.

81 Mettler, F. A., et al. 2008. "Effective Doses in Radiology and Diagnostic Nuclear Medicine: A Catalog." *Radiology* 248(1): 254–63.

82 Whelan, T. J., et al. 2010. "Long-Term Results of Hypofractionated Radiation Therapy for Breast Cancer." *New England Journal of Medicine* 362(6): 513–20.

83 Sze Wai, M., et al. 2002. "Palliation of Metastatic Bone Pain: Single Fraction Versus Multifraction Radiotherapy." *Cochrane Database of Systematic Reviews.* http://dx.doi.org/10.1002/14651858.CD004721.

84 Peters, L. J., et al. 2010. "Critical Impact of Radiotherapy Protocol Compliance and Quality in the Treatment of Advanced Head and Neck Cancer: Results from TROG 02.02." *Journal of Clinical Oncology* 28(18): 2996–3001.

85 Furman et al. 2013. "Gastric Perforation Following Stereotactic Body Radiation."

86 Brunskill, K., et al. 2017. "Does Peer Review of Radiation Plans Impact Clinical Care? A Systematic Review of the Literature." *International Journal of Radiation Oncology, Biology, Physics* 97(1): 27–34.

87 Ford, E., et al. 2011. "WE-C-214-05: A Quantification of the Effectiveness of Standard QA Measures at Preventing Errors in Radiation Therapy and the Promise of In Vivo EPID–Based Portal Dosimetry." *Medical Physics* 38(6): 3808.

88 See Peters et al. 2010. "Critical Impact of Radiotherapy Protocol Compliance." Also: Wuthrick, E. J., et al. 2015. "Institutional Clinical Trial Accrual Volume and Survival of Patients with Head and Neck Cancer." *Journal of Clinical Oncology* 33(2): 156–64; Boero, I. J., et al. 2016. "Importance of Radiation Oncologist Experience Among Patients with Head-and-Neck Cancer Treated with Intensity-Modulated Radiation Therapy." *Journal of Clinical Oncology* 34(7): 684–90; and Chen, Y.-W., et al. 2015. "Association Between Treatment at a High-Volume Facility and Improved Survival for Radiation-Treated Men with High-Risk Prostate Cancer." *International Journal of Radiation Oncology, Biology, Physics* 94(4): 683–90.

89 Peters et al. 2010. "Critical Impact of Radiotherapy Protocol Compliance."

90 Nutting, C. M., et al. 2011. "Parotid-Sparing Intensity Modulated Versus Conventional Radiotherapy in Head and Neck Cancer (PARSPORT): A Phase 3 Multicentre Randomised Controlled Trial." *Lancet Oncology* 12(2): 127–36.

91 Liao, Z. X., et al. 2016. "Bayesian Randomized Trial Comparing Intensity Modulated Radiation Therapy Versus Passively Scattered Proton Therapy for Locally Advanced Non-Small Cell Lung Cancer." *Journal of Clinical Oncology* 34(suppl.; abstr. 8500).

92 DeVita, V. T., and E. Chu. 2008. "A History of Cancer Chemotherapy." *Cancer Research* 68(21): 8643–53.

93 See, for example, Duggan, D. B., et al. 2003. "Randomized Comparison of ABVD and MOPP/ABV Hybrid for the Treatment of Advanced Hodgkin's Disease: Report of an Intergroup Trial." *Journal of Clinical Oncology* 21(4): 607–14.

94 Early Breast Cancer Trialists' Collaborative Group. 2012. "Comparisons Between Different Polychemotherapy Regimens for Early Breast Cancer: Meta-Analyses of Long-Term Outcome Among 100,000 Women in 123 Randomised Trials." *Lancet* 379(9814): 432–44.

95   Blanchard, P., et al. 2011. "Meta-Analysis of Chemotherapy in Head and Neck Cancer (MACH-NC): A Comprehensive Analysis by Tumour Site." *Radiotherapy and Oncology* 100(1): 33–40.

96   Haj Mohammad, N., et al. 2016. "Volume Matters in the Systemic Treatment of Metastatic Pancreatic Cancer: A Population-Based Study in the Netherlands." *Journal of Cancer Research and Clinical Oncology* 142(6): 1353–60.

97   Giri, S., et al. 2015. "Impact of Hospital Volume on Outcomes of Patients Undergoing Chemotherapy for Acute Myeloid Leukemia: A Matched Cohort Study." *Blood* 125(21): 3359–60.

98   Hajage, D., et al. 2011. "External Validation of Adjuvant! Online Breast Cancer Prognosis Tool: Prioritising Recommendations for Improvement." *PLoS One* 6(11): e27446.

99   Tournoux, C., et al. 2006. "Factors Influencing Inclusion of Patients with Malignancies in Clinical Trials." *Cancer* 106(2): 258–70.

100   Hurria, A., et al. 2012. "Senior Adult Oncology." *Journal of the National Comprehensive Cancer Network* 10(2): 162–209.

101   Kass, N., et al. 2008. "Purpose and Benefits of Early Phase Cancer Trials: What Do Oncologists Say? What Do Patients Hear?" *Journal of Empirical Research on Human Research Ethics* 3(3): 57–68.

102   Robert, C., et al. 2015. "Nivolumab in Previously Untreated Melanoma Without *BRAF* Mutation." *New England Journal of Medicine* 372(4): 320–30.

103   Sznol, M., et al. 2013. "Survival and Long-Term Follow-Up of Safety and Response in Patients (Pts) with Advanced Melanoma (MEL) in a Phase I Trial of Nivolumab (Anti-PD-1; BMS-936558; ONO-4538)." *Journal of Clinical Oncology* 31(suppl.; abstr. CRA9006).

104   For two examples, see Druker, B. J., et al. 2001. "Activity of a Specific Inhibitor of the BCR-ABL Tyrosine Kinase in the Blast Crisis of Chronic Myeloid Leukemia and Acute Lymphoblastic Leukemia with the Philadelphia Chromosome." *New England Journal of Medicine* 344(14): 1038–42; and Camidge, D. R., et al. 2012. "Activity and Safety of Crizotinib in Patients with *ALK*-Positive Non-Small-Cell Lung Cancer: Updated Results from a Phase 1 Study." *Lancet Oncology* 13(10): 1011–19.

105 Majumdar, S. R., et al. 2008. "Better Outcomes for Patients Treated at Hospitals That Participate in Clinical Trials." *Archives of Internal Medicine* 168(6): 657–62.

106 Chow, C. J., et al. 2013. "Does Enrollment in Cancer Trials Improve Survival?" *Journal of the American College of Surgeons* 216(4): 774–80.

107 Unger, J. M., et al. 2014. "Comparison of Survival Outcomes Among Cancer Patients Treated in and out of Clinical Trials." *Journal of the National Cancer Institute* 106(3): dju002. http://dx.doi.org/10.1093/jnci /dju002.

108 Peppercorn, J. M., et al. 2004. "Comparison of Outcomes in Cancer Patients Treated Within and Outside Clinical Trials: Conceptual Framework and Structured Review." *Lancet* 363(9405): 263–70.

109 Mayer, D. K., et al. 2014. "American Society of Clinical Oncology Clinical Expert Statement on Cancer Survivorship Care Planning." *Journal of Oncology Practice* 10(6): 345–51.

110 For some background reading on SCPs, see: Mayer, D. K., et al. 2015. "Assuring Quality Cancer Survivorship Care: We've Only Just Begun." *American Society of Clinical Oncology Educational Book*, e583–91; and Hewitt M., S. Greenfield, and E. Stovall, eds. 2005. *From Cancer Patient to Cancer Survivor: Lost in Transition.* Washington, DC: National Academies Press.

111 Birken, S. A., et al. 2014. "Following Through: The Consistency of Survivorship Care Plan Use in United States Cancer Programs." *Journal of Cancer Education* 29(4): 689–97.

112 American College of Surgeons. 2016. "Cancer Program Standards: Ensuring Patient-Centered Care Manual (2016 Edition)." https://www.facs.org/quality%20programs/cancer/coc/standards.

113 Grunfeld, E., et al. 2011. "Evaluating Survivorship Care Plans: Results of a Randomized, Clinical Trial of Patients with Breast Cancer." *Journal of Clinical Oncology* 29(36): 4755–62; and Nicolaije, K. A., et al. 2015. "Impact of an Automatically Generated Cancer Survivorship Care Plan on Patient-Reported Outcomes in Routine Clinical Practice: Longitudinal Outcomes of a Pragmatic, Cluster Randomized Trial." *Journal of Clinical Oncology* 33(31): 3550–59.

114 Smith, T. J., and C. Snyder. 2011. "Is It Time for (Survivorship Care) Plan B?" *Journal of Clinical Oncology* 29(36): 4740–42.

115 Krebber, A. M., et al. 2014. "Prevalence of Depression in Cancer Patients: A Meta-Analysis of Diagnostic Interviews and Self-Report Instruments." *Psycho-Oncology* 23(2): 121–30.

116 Waraich, P., et al. 2004. "Prevalence and Incidence Studies of Mood Disorders: A Systematic Review of the Literature." *Canadian Journal of Psychiatry* 49(2): 124–38.

117 Low, C. A., et al. 2016. "Depressive Symptoms in Patients Scheduled for Hyperthermic Intraperitoneal Chemotherapy with Cytoreductive Surgery: Prospective Associations with Morbidity and Mortality." *Journal of Clinical Oncology* 34(11): 1217–22; Watson, M., et al. 1999. "Influence of Psychological Response on Survival in Breast Cancer: A Population-Based Cohort Study." *Lancet* 354(9187): 1331–33; and Pinquart, M., and P. R. Duberstein. 2010. "Depression and Cancer Mortality: A Meta-Analysis." *Psychological Medicine* 40(11): 1797–810.

118 Mausbach, B. T., and S. A. Irwin. 2016. "Depression and Healthcare Service Utilization in Patients with Cancer." *Psycho-Oncology.* http://dx.doi.org/10.1002/pon.4133.

119 Watson et al. 1999. "Influence of Psychological Response."

120 Pinquart and Duberstein. 2010. "Depression and Cancer Mortality."

121 Toll, B. A., et al. 2013. "Assessing Tobacco Use by Cancer Patients and Facilitating Cessation: An American Association for Cancer Research Policy Statement." *Clinical Cancer Research* 19(8): 1941–48.

122 Ibid.

123 Kwan, M. L., et al. 2010. "Alcohol Consumption and Breast Cancer Recurrence and Survival Among Women with Early-Stage Breast Cancer: The Life After Cancer Epidemiology Study." *Journal of Clinical Oncology* 28(29): 4410–16.

124 Holmes, M. D. 2010. "Challenge of Balancing Alcohol Intake." *Journal of Clinical Oncology* 28(29): 4403–4.

125 For these statistics, see American Cancer Society. 2016. "Cancer Facts & Figures 2016." http://www.cancer.org/research/cancerfactsstatistics /cancerfactsfigures2016/. See also American Cancer Society. 2011. "Global Cancer Facts & Figures 2nd Edition." http://www.cancer.org/ acs/groups/content/@epidemiologysurveilance/documents/document/ acspc-027766.pdf.

126 Palma, D. A., et al. 2014. "The Oligometastatic State: Separating Truth from Wishful Thinking." *National Reviews Clinical Oncology* 11(9): 549–57.

127 See, for example: Andrews, D. W., et al. 2004. "Whole Brain Radiation Therapy with or Without Stereotactic Radiosurgery Boost for Patients with One to Three Brain Metastases: Phase III Results of the RTOG 9508 Randomised Trial." *Lancet* 363(9422): 1665–72; Patchell, R. A., et al. 1990. "A Randomized Trial of Surgery in the Treatment of Single Metastases to the Brain." *New England Journal of Medicine* 322(8): 494–500; and Soran, A., et al. 2016. "A Randomized Controlled Trial Evaluating Resection of the Primary Breast Tumor in Women Presenting with De Novo Stage IV Breast Cancer: Turkish Study (Protocol MF07–01)." *Journal of Clinical Oncology* 34(suppl.; abstr. 1005).

128 Choosing Wisely. "Care at the End of Life for Advanced Cancer Patients." http://www.choosingwisely.org/patient-resources/care-at-the-end-of -life-for-advanced-cancer-patients/.

129 Chen, R. C., et al. 2016. "Aggressive Care at the End-of-Life for Younger Patients with Cancer: Impact of ASCO's Choosing Wisely Campaign." *Journal of Clinical Oncology* 34(suppl.; abstr. LBA10033).

130 For more details on what palliative care comprises, see "WHO Definition of Palliative Care" at http://www.who.int/cancer/palliative/definition/en/.

131 LeBlanc, T. W., et al. 2016. "Discussing the Evidence for Upstream Palliative Care in Improving Outcomes in Advanced Cancer." *American Society for Clinical Oncology Education Book* 35: e534–38.

132 Ibid.

133 Fabrice, D., et al. 2016. "Overall Survival in Patients with Lung Cancer Using a Web-Application-Guided Follow-Up Compared to Standard Modalities: Results of Phase III Randomized Trial." *Journal of Clinical Oncology* 34 (suppl.; abstr. LBA9006).

134 See LeBlanc et al. 2016. "Discussing the Evidence for Upstream Palliative Care"; and Back, A. L., et al. 2014. "Clinician Roles in Early Integrated Palliative Care for Patients with Advanced Cancer: A Qualitative Study." *Journal of Palliative Medicine* 17(11): 1244–48.

135 Pirl, W. F., et al. 2012. "Depression and Survival in Metastatic Non-Small-Cell Lung Cancer: Effects of Early Palliative Care." *Journal of Clinical Oncology* 30(12): 1310–15.

136 Sweeney, C. J., et al. 2015. "Chemohormonal Therapy in Metastatic Hormone-Sensitive Prostate Cancer." *New England Journal of Medicine* 373(8): 737–46.

137 Pignon, J. P., et al. 2008. "Lung Adjuvant Cisplatin Evaluation: A Pooled Analysis by the LACE Collaborative Group." *Journal of Clinical Oncology* 26(21): 3552–59.

138 Early Breast Cancer Trialists' Collaborative Group. 2012. "Comparisons Between Different Polychemotherapy Regimens for Early Breast Cancer: Meta-Analyses of Long-Term Outcome Among 100,000 Women in 123 Randomised Trials." *Lancet* 379(9814): 432–44.

139 See Druker, B. J., et al. 2001. "Efficacy and Safety of a Specific Inhibitor of the BCR-ABL Tyrosine Kinase in Chronic Myeloid Leukemia." *New England Journal of Medicine* 344(14): 1031–37; and O'Brien, S. G., et al. 2003. "Imatinib Compared with Interferon and Low-Dose Cytarabine for Newly Diagnosed Chronic-Phase Chronic Myeloid Leukemia." *New England Journal of Medicine* 348(11): 994–1004.

140 Robert, C., et al. 2015. "Nivolumab in Previously Untreated Melanoma Without *BRAF* Mutation." *New England Journal of Medicine* 372(4): 320–30.

141 Ornish, D., et al. 2005. "Intensive Lifestyle Changes May Affect the Progression of Prostate Cancer." *Journal of Urolology* 174(3): 1065–69.

142 Chlebowski, R. T., et al. 2006. "Dietary Fat Reduction and Breast Cancer Outcome: Interim Efficacy Results from the Women's Intervention Nutrition Study." *Journal of the National Cancer Institute* 98(24): 1767–76.

143 See Prentice, R. L., et al. 2006. "Low-Fat Dietary Pattern and Risk of Invasive Breast Cancer: The Women's Health Initiative Randomized Controlled Dietary Modification Trial." *Journal of the American Medical Association* 295(6): 629–42; and Beresford, S. A., et al. 2006. "Low-Fat Dietary Pattern and Risk of Colorectal Cancer: The Women's Health Initiative Randomized Controlled Dietary Modification Trial." *Journal of the American Medical Association* 295(6): 643–54.

144   Van Patten, C. L., J. G. de Boer, and E. S. Tomlinson Guns. 2008. "Diet and Dietary Supplement Intervention Trials for the Prevention of Prostate Cancer Recurrence: A Review of the Randomized Controlled Trial Evidence." *Journal of Urology* 180(6): 2314–22; and Tramm, R., A. L. McCarthy, and P. Yates. 2011. "Dietary Modification for Women After Breast Cancer Treatment: A Narrative Review." *European Journal of Cancer Care* 20(3): 294–304.

145   Meyerhardt, J. A., et al. 2007. "Association of Dietary Patterns with Cancer Recurrence and Survival in Patients with Stage III Colon Cancer." *Journal of the American Medical Association* 298(7): 754–64.

146   Padayatty, S. J., et al. 2003. "Vitamin C as an Antioxidant: Evaluation of Its Role in Disease Prevention." *Journal of the American College of Nutrition* 22(1): 18–35.

147   Fuchs-Tarlovsky, V. 2013. "Role of Antioxidants in Cancer Therapy." *Nutrition* 29(1): 15–21.

148   Unlu, A., et al. 2016. "High-Dose Vitamin C and Cancer." *Journal of Oncological Science* 1: 10–12. See also Fuchs-Tarlovsy. 2013. "Role of Antioxidants."

149   Alpha-Tocopherol Beta Carotene Cancer Prevention Study Group. 1994. "The Effect of Vitamin E and Beta Carotene on the Incidence of Lung Cancer and Other Cancers in Male Smokers." *New England Journal of Medicine* 330(15): 1029–35.

150   National Health and Medical Research Council. 2015. "NHMRC Statement on Homeopathy and NHMRC Information Paper: Evidence on the Effectiveness of Homeopathy for Treating Health Conditions." https://www.nhmrc.gov.au/guidelines-publications/cam02.

151   Elvis, A. M., and J. S. Ekta. 2011. "Ozone Therapy: A Clinical Review." *Journal of Natural Science, Biology, and Medicine* 2(1): 66–70.

152   Risberg, T., et al. 2003. "Does Use of Alternative Medicine Predict Survival from Cancer?" *European Journal of Cancer* 39(3): 372–77.

153   Yun, Y. H., et al. 2013. "Effect of Complementary and Alternative Medicine on the Survival and Health-Related Quality of Life Among Terminally Ill Cancer Patients: A Prospective Cohort Study." *Annals of Oncology* 24(2): 489–94.

154 Mailankody, S., and V. Prasad. 2015. "Five Years of Cancer Drug Approvals: Innovation, Efficacy, and Costs." *JAMA Oncology* 1(4): 539–40.

155 Kantarjian, H., et al. 2014. "High Cancer Drug Prices in the United States: Reasons and Proposed Solutions." *Journal of Oncology Practice* 10(4): e208–11.

156 Lundh, A., et al. 2012. "Industry Sponsorship and Research Outcome." *Cochrane Database of Systematic Reviews.* http://dx.doi.org/10.1002/1465 1858.MR000033.pub2.

157 Lexchin, J., et al. 2003. "Pharmaceutical Industry Sponsorship and Research Outcome and Quality: Systematic Review." *British Medical Journal* 326(7400): 1167–70.

158 De Angelis, C., et al. 2004. "Clinical Trial Registration: A Statement from the International Committee of Medical Journal Editors." *New England Journal of Medicine* 351(12): 1250–51.

159 Taichman, D. B., et al. 2016. "Sharing Clinical Trial Data: A Proposal from the International Committee of Medical Journal Editors." *New England Journal of Medicine* 374(4): 384–86.

160 Agrawal, S., N. Brennan, and P. Budetti. 2013. "The Sunshine Act: Effects on Physicians." *New England Journal of Medicine* 368(22): 2054–57.

161 American Cancer Society. "Cancer Facts & Figures 2016." http://www .cancer.org/research/cancerfactsstatistics/cancerfactsfigures2016/.

162 Canadian Cancer Society. 2015. "Canadian Cancer Statistics." www .cancer.ca/~/media/cancer.ca/CW/cancer%20information/cancer%20 101/Canadian%20cancer%20statistics/Canadian-Cancer-Statistics -2015-EN.pdf.

About the Author

David Palma, MD, PhD, is a radiation oncologist and cancer researcher focusing on the treatment of lung, head and neck, and metastatic cancers. He holds advanced degrees from Harvard University, the VU University in Amsterdam, and Western University in Canada. Palma has published more than one hundred scientific research articles, and has won several awards for academics and teaching. He lives in Canada with his wife Cheryl Smits—a family doctor—and their three children. He is an avid marathon runner and Ironman triathlete.

Foreword writer **Anthony Zietman, MD**, is Shipley Professor of Radiation Oncology at Harvard Medical School, and former president of the American Society for Radiation Oncology (ASTRO). He is chief editor of the *International Journal of Radiation Oncology Biology Physics*—one of the world's leading radiation oncology journals—and is a trustee of the American Board of Radiology.

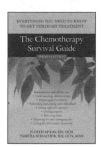
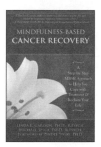
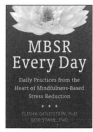
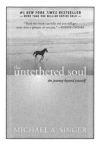
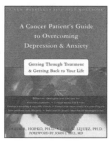
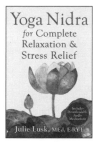
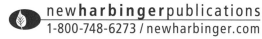 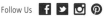